Insights from a Sixty-Four-Year Case of Anorexia Nervosa

This volume offers rare insight into an enduring case of anorexia nervosa in a female patient and details the approaches to treatment taken by psychotherapists throughout the 64 year period 1938-2002.

Through discussion and analysis of clinical notes and transcripts, Lipsitt traces the course of the patient's illness to consider the centrality of the mother–daughter relationship and to highlight aspects of constancy and change in the illness over time. Particular attention is paid to shifts and progress in understanding and treatment of anorexia nervosa, and consideration is also given to how contemporary treatment might differ in view of more recent advances in cognitive behavioral approaches. Offering an innovative approach toward addressing the transgenerational perspective of women's experiences of eating disorders, this book provides material for a range of professionals to discuss the nature of the disorder and the pros and cons of different treatment approaches.

An original take on the relationship dynamics and perspectives of anorexia sufferers, this volume will be of interest to students, faculty and scholars with an interest in studying eating disorders and their treatment approaches, including psychoanalytic psychotherapy.

Don R. Lipsitt, M.D., is Professor of Psychiatry (part-time) at Harvard Medical School and Associate in Psychiatry, Beth Israel Deaconess Medical Center, Boston, MA, USA.

Routledge Research in Women's Mental Health

This series offers an international forum for original and innovative research being conducted across the field of Mental Health. Titles in the series are empirically or theoretically informed and explore a range of dynamic and timely issues and emerging topics with particular relevance to women's mental health. The series is aimed at upper-level and post-graduate students, researchers and research students as well as academics and scholars.

Recent titles in the series:

Understanding Complex Trauma and Post-Traumatic Growth in Survivors of Sex Trafficking
Foregrounding Women's Voices for Effective Care and Prevention
Heather Evans

Pregnancy-Related Anxiety
Theory, Research, and Practice
Edited by Rachel Dryer and Robyn Brunton

Insights from a Sixty-Four-Year Case of Anorexia Nervosa
Constancy and Change in Symptoms and Treatment
Don R. Lipsitt

For more information about this series, please visit https://www.routledge.com/Routledge-Research-in-Womens-Mental-Health/book-series/RRWMH.

Insights from a Sixty-Four-Year Case of Anorexia Nervosa

Constancy and Change in Symptoms and Treatment

Don R. Lipsitt

Routledge
Taylor & Francis Group
NEW YORK AND LONDON

First published 2023
by Routledge
605 Third Avenue, New York, NY 10158, USA

and by Routledge
4 Park Square, Milton Park, Abingdon, Oxon, OX14 4RN, UK

Routledge is an imprint of the Taylor & Francis Group, an informa business.

ISBN: 978-1-032-07767-3 (hbk)
ISBN: 978-1-032-07769-7 (pbk)
ISBN: 978-1-003-20869-3 (ebk)

DOI: 10.4324/9781003208693

Typeset in Sabon
by SPi Technologies India Pvt Ltd (Straive)

To my late brother, Lew, whose prodigious revelations of infant behavior have made us all more knowledgeable and respectful of what it is to be human

and

To my dear late colleague and long-time friend, Robert Eisendrath, who made psychiatry a serious profession without sacrificing a place for fun

Contents

Figures

Preamble

The impetus for this book arose from a series of sheer happenstance. I had written a contribution to the 50th anniversary issue of the journal *Psychosomatic Medicine* in 1989 that included an abbreviated history of a young woman with anorexia. Her story included an interview in 1938 by Dr. Felix Deutsch, a pioneer psychoanalyst who reputedly coined the term "psychosomatic medicine." My former residency chief in 1956 at Albert Einstein Medical Center, Dr. Milton Rosenbaum, during his own psychiatric residency in 1938 at Massachusetts General (MGH) and McLean Hospitals (McLH) had been a contemporary of Dr. Deutsch and himself a pioneer of psychosomatic medicine. Seeing my journal article, Rosenbaum recognized remarks by Deutsch and me, and sent the paper to his friend and one-time co-fellow, Dr. John Romano, who had been a psychiatry/neurology trainee at Boston's Peter Bent Brigham Hospital around the same time that Deutsch had interviewed the patient. This, quite unexpectedly, elicited a letter from Romano to me, accompanied remarkably by a small sheaf of typed notes Romano had saved after he too had interviewed the same patient at Boston hospitals in 1938–1942. (During that time, his training had included a brief encounter with psychoanalysis at the Boston Psychoanalytic Institute (BPSI) as a Freud Fellow. Rosenbaum and Romano found kinship in their common interest in psychosomatic medicine.)

And so, with mounting material about this one patient with whom I too had become acquainted, it seemed of value to assemble these data with an updated report of her lengthy course—probably the longest outcome report of an anorexic patient, hence, the birth of this monograph—about a woman diagnosed with anorexia nervosa in 1938. I encountered her in 1961 when I was asked to consult on her during an emergency admission to Boston's Beth Israel Hospital (BIH). I continued to meet with her and followed her course until she died in 2002. What follows is a longitudinal account of her medical journey over a period of more than 60 years.

This account does not intend an exhaustive review of the abundant research and therapeutic interventions that have accompanied the history of anorexia nervosa, but rather the story of one woman from the time of diagnosis as an adolescent to demise 64 years later. It is the wish of the author to add insights to an understanding of a ravishing disease with notoriously poor outcomes to date.

Acknowledgments[1]

Writing is a lonely enterprise. Being asocial helps a bit, as does a pandemic. But the wizardry of modern technology keeps me attached to the external world along with major assists from computer gurus grandson Jonah and nephew Daniel. It has allowed me to be the beneficiary of the interest, support, love and caring of many, as they accompany me on the path I have taken. There is, of course, the devotion of my two remarkable sons, Eric and Steven, and their equally remarkable wives, Brenda and Mara, without whose presence and encouragement I could not have kept on. And my dear companion, Betty Grossman, not only has provided a life-support system but is a walking thesaurus. Drs. Jonathan Blumberg and Lisa Weissmann, nurse extraordinaire Donna Gallagher and ducklings Erika, Rachel and Vicki have been too much a presence in my life but indispensable in keeping me at my laptop while the job is being done. The spirit of my best friend, Merna, joins me daily at the computer. Luci's cleaning squad, Molly's cookery and even the condo concierges keep the system whirring. With the loss of brother Lew, the Lipsitt Five is no more, but calls from senior brother Paul and junior brothers Cyrus and Peter are reassuring. And inquiries from cousin age-mate Reba Mirsky Goodman is confirmatory that we are both still here! Old college friend Sydney Wolfe Cohen, gone too soon, premier indexer of previous work, could not oblige this time, but we continued indexing past memories until the end. Without Ms. B graciously allowing me into her life, this story would not exist. And the same is true if my parents, Anna and Joseph, had not brought me into theirs.

Then, of course, there is the endless circle of invisible but very present editors, overseen by Alice Salt, who work their magic to bring the entire enterprise to its glorious (?) conclusion. I hope we all revel in its product.

What a joyful isolation!

1 I wish to express special thanks to Drs. Betty J. Grossman and Eric D. Lipsitt for their thoughtful review of chapters and suggestions. Mistakes and omissions are, of course, entirely my own.

1 Introduction

> Mr. Duke's daughter in St. Mary Axe, in the year 1684, and the Eighteenth Year of her Age, in the month of July, fell into a total suppression of her Monthly Courses from a multitude of Passions and Cares of her Mind, but without any symptoms of the Green-Sickness following upon it.
>
> – Richard Morton, *Phthisiologia*, 1689

Note on Eating

Although abnormalities of menstruation attracted physicians' attention as a first concern 300 years ago in anorexic young women, "among the 'multitude of passions and cares of [the] mind'" noted by Morton in 1689, eating is most certainly one of the earliest life-sustaining activities, later becoming ritualized, socialized and regulated. Its meaningful connection with mother (or her surrogates) is developmentally crucial to what a child/person may become. Relationship to mother, her breast (or substitute) and affective tie will begin the process of the child's maturation and perhaps has vital meaning for a lifetime.

Figuring prominently in processes of attachment and separation (Bowlby, 1969), the oral phase of development, with its highly charged valence from the first moments of life, also captured Sigmund Freud's interest in the child's psychosexual development (Freud, 1905). Although, for many reasons, Freud's treatment of Dora was considered a failure and overlooked the mother's influence on the daughter's behavior, it did reveal "typical derivatives of adolescent conflicts and defenses," so important in understanding the young anorexic's illness as well as countertransference reactions of therapists toward these patients (Jennings, 1986). Although Freud did not address anorexia nervosa per se, he did take note of Dora's eating behavior and her disgust with food as "hysterical symptoms" that could be "traced to regression from adolescent sexuality to forbidden infantile wishes" (Deutsch, 1957; Sayers, 1988).

The experience of eating may be pleasurable or even at times distasteful. Individuals learn gustatory nature, the goodness or badness, and the power of food, not only as a nutritional essential but also as something

DOI: 10.4324/9781003208693-1

that can be manipulated to exert control over oneself and others. Hunger strikes have been known for ages as a way of influencing administrative, governmental or political change. A reaction of disgust at certain foods is not an uncommon natural experience.

Within the family constellation, food becomes a central focus of communal life and has strong connotations of love when proffered or withheld in daily child–parent relations. Many researchers who have studied mother–infant relations stress the formative nature of this behavior (Brazelton et al., 1974; Hinds & Lipsitt, 1982; Kagan & Zentner, 1996; Winnicott, 1960).

> It's impossible to observe a human mother and her infant interacting with one another directly after birth, without realizing that something exceedingly important is going on between the two of them. They look at each other, spar, reciprocate gestures and behaviors... and that is the scene out of which that child's humanity will grow.
>
> (Hinds & Lipsitt, 1982, p. 22)

"Infancy is in large part a rehearsal for the future" (p. 30).

Certainly, mothers need not be perfect, but in Winnicott's description they must be a "good enough mother" who can provide an environment that will nourish a child physically, emotionally, gastronomically as well as socially. In Belsky's model of parenting, the infant "needs a 'goodness-of-fit' between infant and maternal temperaments" (Belsky, 1984). In situations where mother's concerns are more with herself, the infant will suffer the repercussions.

The patient with anorexia nervosa learns exquisitely how to turn the act of eating to her or his own purposes and is effectively capable of weaponizing the process in interactions with parents. This monograph recounts the role of eating in a turbulent mother–daughter relationship extending over decades, the results persisting virtually (symbolically) even after the mother's demise. This patient's anorexia nervosa was diagnosed in 1938, and this story traces her medical-psychiatric journey from adolescence to late adulthood.

As individuals benefit from the remarkable successes of science and medicine through most of the previous century, new findings in heart disease, hypertension, cancer, infectious and immunologic diseases, diabetes, and many others have given promise to many who have previously lived in despair. Sadly, there remain a few illnesses for which so little progress has been made, as research toils vigorously to achieve improved outcomes. Dementing illnesses, other neurologic diseases and some cancers are the most resistant. Anorexia nervosa, a multisystem, treatment-resistant and often fatal disease, joins that group with persistently poor outcome. Declared by some as "the paradigmatic psychosomatic disease" (Kaufman & Heiman, 1964), it has many social vectors and varied physiologic, anatomic and mental consequences and puzzling symptomatology, posing a major clinical challenge to early and accurate diagnosis.

Opportunities for long-term observation of treatments and outcomes rarely present themselves in medicine. Patients seek alternate services, move or die. Physicians-in-training transition to the next level and transfer patients to successive possibly naive clinicians. Practicing physicians may make extensive patient notes that are often not preserved. Physicians retire or die; records are destroyed or lost.

Thus, in the case described here, the extensive notes of a patient's therapeutic journey from age 19 into her much later years provide a rare occasion to observe changes in treatment attitudes, therapeutics, physician observations, course of illness and long-term outcome. What follows is not another article, volume, textbook or personal memoir. Rather, it is an account of a woman whose story spans more than 60 years since first diagnosis in 1938 to the time she died in 2002. The intent is not only to illustrate the "dynamics" of a single case but also to highlight the relative consistency over the years, in exceptional detail, of how the patient interacted with consecutive therapists, who possibly subscribed to different theoretical models of the disease. Clinical notes also reveal constant threads of symptoms, behavior and interpersonal relations, especially with the mother but also with nurses and other personnel. The story casts light and shadow on how a single case of anorexia and its treatment evolved in the 20th century.

The story is one of struggles and distress of a mother and daughter confronting the disease and each other as they attempt to achieve some semblance of a satisfying life. In addition to a case summary as recorded in the late 1930s and early 1940s, detailed notes of interviews by subsequent therapists are included to give a flavor of the patient's style of interacting. These notes are recreated from original meticulous clinical records. Therapy as described in those notes does not expound specific therapeutic theories, although therapists themselves were psychiatrists and psychoanalysts; treatment seemed largely supportive and ventilatory. Progress notes over the years suggest that the patient was "not suitable for a more dynamic therapy." First seen in 1938 by Dr. John Waller, then Dr. Felix Deutsch, followed by Dr. John Romano, she had briefer contacts with other therapists from time to time. Finally, from 1961, she met episodically with me until her death in 2002.

Every measure is taken to disguise identification of the patient, her family and her doctors, except in those instances where the author has been granted permission. The story involves scores of physicians, including psychiatrists, social workers, nurses and other health-care professionals, most of whom are now deceased. During her lifetime, the patient signed several consents to permit review of her records with educational objectives, including publication.

References

Belsky, J. (1984). The determinants of parenting: a process model. *Child Development*, 55(1), 83–96.

Bowlby, J. (1969). *Attachment and Loss I: Attachment*. New York: Basic Books.

Brazelton, T.B., Koslowski, B., & Main, M. (1974). The origins of reciprocity: The early mother-infant interaction. In M. Lewis & L.A. Rosenblum (Eds.) *The Effect of the Infant on Its Caregiver*. New York: Wiley Interscience.

Deutsch, F. (1957). A footnote to Freud's "Fragment of an analysis of a case of hysteria". *Psychoanalytic Quarterly*, 26(2), 159–167.

Freud, S. (1905). Three essays on the theory of sexuality. *Standard Edition*, 7, 125–245.

Hinds, K., & Lipsitt L.P. (1982). Finding out why kids are the way they are. *Brown Monthly Alumni Magazine*, 83(4), 22–31.

Jennings, J.J. (1986). The revival of "Dora": advances in psychoanalytic theory and technique. *Journal of the American Psychoanalytic Association*, 34(3), 607–635.

Kagan, J., & Zentner, M. (1996). Early childhood predictors of adult psychopathology. *Harvard Review of Psychiatry*, 3(6), 341–350.

Kaufman, M.R., & Heiman, M. (Eds.) (1964). *Evolution of Psychosomatic Concepts: Anorexia Nervosa: A Paradigm*. New York: International Universities Press, Inc.

Morton, R. (1689). *Phthisiologia, or a Treatise of Consumption*. London: S. Smith & B. Walford.

Sayers, J. (1988). Anorexia, psychoanalysis, and feminism: fantasy and reality. *Journal of Adolescence*, 11(4), 361–371.

Winnicott, D.W. (1960). The theory of the parent-infant relationship. *International Journal of Psychoanalysis*, 41, 585–595.

2 Origins of the Diagnosis of Anorexia Nervosa

Historians have traced eating disorders back thousands of years, and some instances of "eating disorders" include religious practices of fasting and restrictive eating in a quest for thinness. Anorexia nervosa in some form is one of the longest known medical and psychiatric disorders.

Richard Morton (1689) reported an early case, which he called "consumption," thought to be related to tuberculosis and referred to as "*phthisis nervosa*," attributed to "a want of appetite" or "studying too hard" (Ryle, 1936). Early reports referred to "chlorosis" or the "green sickness," treated as a kind of anemia (Loudon, 1980, 1984). Literature on this topic emphasizes the impact of social circumstances on the naming of a disease, and chlorosis was seen as a common diagnosis in the 1870s and 1880s, essentially disappearing after the First World War and perhaps replaced by "anorexia nervosa" (Blumberg, 1982; Theriot, 1988). Medical advertisements for remedies for chlorosis populated medical journals of the times (Figure 2.1).

Less attention was paid to the association of chlorosis with eating disorders than to perturbations of menstruation in early 19th-century medicine. It was known, for example, that fears of pregnancy could delay menstruation or cause extensive menorrhea (Kaufman & Heiman, 1964, p. 25; Raciborski, 1865).

An illness is not officially acknowledged until it is named. How an illness comes to be named is a sometimes curious and interesting process in itself (Shorter, 1992, p. 2) as the history of chlorosis vividly portrays. Rudolf Virchow, in 1848, had asked "do we not always find the diseases of the populace traceable to defects in society?" (p. 2). It is as though a series of "mystifying" cases over time coalesce into an organized picture or syndrome, at which point the need to share clinical information of diagnosis and treatment leads to naming of the disease. It is much like the sequence in a Marx Brothers film when Chico is playing around on the piano and Groucho says to Chico "When you get near a tune, play it." It took a couple of hundred years for the name anorexia nervosa to gain sustainability and permanence.

DOI: 10.4324/9781003208693-2

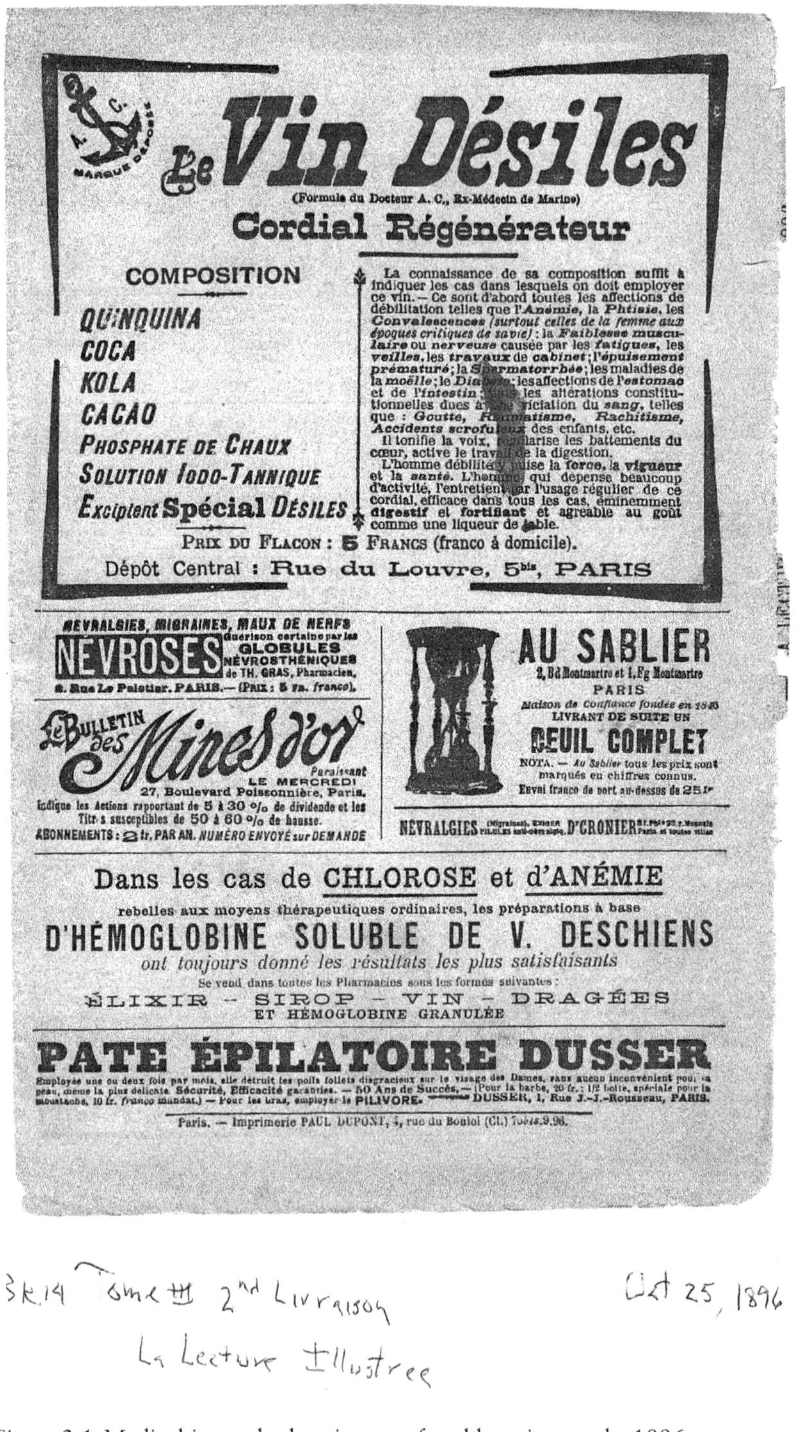

Figure 2.1 Medical journal advertisement for chlorosis remedy, 1896.

As references to chlorosis and the green sickness faded, the named disease appeared in the later 1870s, when accounts by Sir William Gull (1874) and Ernest-Charles Lasègue (1873) independently described cases of self-starvation. Lasègue, like Freud, had begun his career with a strong interest in philosophy before pursuing studies in psychiatry, perhaps accounting for greater interest than that of his colleague Gull in the psychological and physiological aspects of anorexia; Gull took a more traditional medical approach to the disease. Based on eight cases, Lasègue's classic paper *De l'Anorexie Hysterique* appeared in 1873, about 5 years after Gull had presented his findings on anorexia to the British Medical Association at Oxford, first calling it *apepsia hysterica*, then *anorexia hysterica* and finally *anorexia nervosa*, the name persisting to this time. Though clearly identified with naming the disease, Gull's fame was centered more on his investment in the notorious case of Jack the Ripper. Both Lasègue and Gull emphasized the importance of family relations in the origin and sustaining of the disease.

By the late 1800s and early 1900s, the importance of a careful assessment of personality began to enter the practice of both medicine and psychiatry, strongly influenced by the psychobiological teaching and writing of Adolf Meyer (Lief, 1948) at Johns Hopkins, with whom Hilde Bruch, one of the early anorexia experts, later studied.

Early Treatments

Treatment approaches have varied, depending on theories of etiology and therapeutics at the time (Lipsitt, 1989). Success has been scant and outcome studies consistently report a relatively high mortality rate hovering around 10%, the highest of any psychiatric illness (Arcelus et al., 2011). It is a disease primarily of women.

The fact that most observed cases of anorexia nervosa occurred around puberty encouraged etiologic conceptualizations that the illness may be related to sexual maturational processes and "romantic" interests (Kluck et al., 2018). Interest in this perplexing "hysterical" illness piqued with the beginnings of psychoanalysis. Eating disorders were seen in one aspect associated with attempts at avoiding the anxiety of sexual intimacy.

In 1964, M. Ralph Kaufman and Marcel Heiman published their book *Evolution of Psychosomatic Concepts: Anorexia Nervosa: A Paradigm* (Kaufman & Heiman, 1964). It was not lost on them that the history of the disease, with its physiological, endocrinological, emotional, neurological and other system involvements, could represent *par excellence* the complex integration of mind–body systems, the study of which was the early mission of the newly founded American Psychosomatic Society and its journal *Psychosomatic Medicine* (1939–1942). Referred to by Kaufman and Heiman as a "paradigmatic psychosomatic illness," anorexia, though less prevalent than most eating disorders, attracted widespread interest because of its elusive etiology and high mortality. As psychosomatic medicine evolved, so have treatments of anorexia. For decades, debate has ensued over the proprietary designation of psychosomatic medicine as a medical or psychiatric specialty. Evidence of the fragmented approach to anorexia is reflected in the broad spectrum of specialties concerned with the disease. As noted by Vigersky (1977), anorexia nervosa is

> of interest to psychiatrists because of its psychology and perceptual abnormalities; to endocrinologists because of its hypothalamic-pituitary-end organ dysfunction; to gynecologists because it frequently presents as secondary amenorrhea; to pediatricians because it often occurs in pre-teenagers and it appears to be a reversal of puberty; and to internists of varied subspecialties because of its protean manifestations and complications. For basic scientists, it serves as a model for the study of the effects of malnutrition, for the investigation of neurogenic amines, and for the understanding of factors such as critical body mass and hypothalamic function. Finally, it presents a major therapeutic challenge that has yet to be successfully met.
>
> (Vigersky, 1977, p. v)

I would add that family therapists of all denominations have a vital preoccupation with the complex dynamics of family relationships and their impact on the onset and course of anorexia. The fact that the illness occurs around puberty and involves attitudes about sexuality encouraged psychoanalysts to apply psychoanalytic theory to attempts at understanding the disease, citing Freud's early postulation of sexual development through oral, anal and phallic stages, including a major focus on oral aspects of eating behavior. Thus, fantasies of oral impregnation through eating conferred symbolic meaning on objects like milk, breast, penis and feces. Even with psychoanalytic interest, Freud nevertheless warned against treating anorexia psychoanalytically because life-threatening physiological elements required urgent *physical* treatment (Sayers, 1988).

A "Wholeness" Approach

The concepts of biopsychosocial medicine proposed by theorists like Ludwig von Bertalanffy (1968) and George Engel (1980) advocated models of collaborative approaches to treatment that fostered new perspectives for clinical practitioners to embrace social aspects of family structure, psychological and physical factors in understanding and diagnosing all illness.

The book edited by Kaufman and Heiman includes reproductions of the early reports of Gull, Lasègue and the Mount Sinai Study Group on anorexia nervosa; an example of one of the earliest psychoanalytic treatments of an anorexic woman; and the case history reported in the journal *Psychosomatic Medicine* by John Waller, Kaufman and Felix Deutsch (1940). Curiously, Kaufman and Heiman's book contains a single bibliographic but no text reference to Bruch. Similarly absent is Flanders Dunbar's (1935) meticulously recorded "all psychosomatic references" from 1910 to 1933 (published in 1938 with mostly reviews of the German literature) without mention of anorexia.

In 1973, Basic Books published Bruch's voluminous reference text *Eating Disorders: Obesity, Anorexia and the Person Within*, considered at the time the definitive work on the treatment of the stubborn and potentially fatal disease anorexia nervosa, although reference to its importance had appeared in the literature previously (Crisp, 1968; Frazier, 1963). Earlier (1963), without much notice, at least one report of the "crisis" of anorexia surfaced when Dr. Shervert Frazier, medical director of McLean Hospital in Belmont, Massachusetts, gave a presentation on the disease to the 39th meeting of the Central Neuropsychiatric Association. An article in the November 18, 1963 issue of *Medical Tribune* (p. 5) headlined Frazier's talk "*Anorexia Nervosa Held to be Medical Crisis*." McLean Hospital was known for treating long-term cases who were often refractory to previous treatments. Frazier described the course and treatment of 39 patients with diagnosed anorexia, describing three peak periods of onset: prepubertal, with best outcomes; adolescence, the sickest, and older than 25 with development of chronicity. Most important features included disturbance of body image, disturbance of perception of internal or visceral state, lack of autonomy, and feeling ineffective or useless. Ten percent of the studied patients were habitual water imbibers, three fourths of cases had a "nagging mother" pattern, 12 were unimproved after hospitalization and treatment and 11 were markedly improved. In 1970, Frazier published an excellent review on anorexia nervosa in *Hospital Medicine* (p. 5), stating "these emaciated patients, suffering from lack of affection and severe emotional isolation, utilize the pursuit of thinness as a weapon in the struggle for control of family members" (Frazier, 1970, p. 60). There were no parades, no walks-for-anorexia, and no major fund-raising activities for this crisis. There was, however, a rare three-site research study sponsored by the National Institute of Mental Health (NIMH) in 1975, investigating the benefits of behavior therapy as treatment for anorexia (Eckert et al., 1979; Halmi, Powers & Cunningham, 1975). Positive reinforcements were used to encourage weight gain, but results were disappointing. Behavior therapy yielded no better results than regular milieu (ward) therapy.

Interest in the subject brought forth a more popularized version of Bruch's book in 1978, titled *The Golden Cage: The Enigma of Anorexia Nervosa*. Although anorexia nervosa represented one of the most intractable and mortal diseases known, research interest lagged until around 1980s, when there was an abundance of exploratory activity.

Bruch was a German-born American psychoanalyst who emigrated to New York City in 1934 to escape war clouds gathering in Europe. Beginning her career as a pediatrician, she pursued interest in obesity in children and received a Josiah Macy, Jr. Foundation fellowship in 1937. After additional psychiatric and psychoanalytic training at the Johns Hopkins University Phipps Clinic, she became curious about the nature of the "skinny disease," anorexia nervosa, although she later rejected much of psychoanalytic speculation about the etiology of the disease. She saw her first case of anorexia nervosa in 1942 as a resident at the Phipps Psychiatric Clinic (Bruch, 1973, p. 233).

After two years in Baltimore, she returned to New York's Columbia University, was appointed professor in 1959, and opened a private practice for the treatment of eating disorders. By 1964, she had accepted a full-time professorship at Baylor College of Medicine and remained there for the rest of her career. (Besides being highly esteemed for her clinical acumen, she was known as the "quirky doctor" with a Rolls Royce, perhaps a personality characteristic that made her appealing to young patients.)

With astute observations, Bruch recognized the many attitudes around eating that were rooted in family patterns as well as various symbolic meanings of food throughout the child's developmental process. Trained fundamentally in dyadic models of treatment, Bruch nonetheless recognized early that parents and family dynamics entered prominently into the picture of anorexia, the "relentless pursuit of thinness." Psychoanalytic insights were of great relevance to understanding attitudes toward food in the maturing child but not of treatment.

Not since the latter part of the 19th century had ideas about anorexia changed very much. Mostly regarded as a "medical" disease, it was first thought to be related to entities like hypopituitarism, tuberculosis or Simmonds' disease or dismissed as "some kind of psychiatric disease" like schizophrenia, depression or hysteria. Medical history is rife with such instances: when faced with a "puzzling" or "undiagnosable" disease, medicine turns to psychiatry for help, a trend that prevails in medical practice.

Death of Karen Anne Carpenter

Sometimes the revelations of a public figure have greater impact than those of science. Such was the 1983 death of the popular American singer, drummer and musician Karen Anne Carpenter from cardiac ravages of anorexia nervosa. Her story catalyzed profound media interest in the disease. Early in life, she had been very active, dancing, singing, and playing baseball with brothers and others. She began the vigorous activity of drumming at a very young age.

She was only 32 when she died, and her story touched women of her generation, especially those with eating disorders. Early precursors of disease likely were obscured by her skills as a musician. Though a small woman, she began to feel uncomfortably heavy, adopted a weight-loss diet and dropped to 91 pounds in 1973. Her relationship with her parents was troublesome. She acknowledged her illness and sought psychotherapy; but, advised that treatment would take at least 3 years, she downplayed it in favor of her dedication to a musical career. A rocky marriage was punctuated with disagreements about raising a family and excessive use of emetics, laxatives and thyroid medication. Others began to take notice of her illness, especially her co-performing brother Richard. Hospitalized at Lenox Hill Hospital, she regained a bit of weight, but the cardiac sequelae of starvation and malnutrition impeded full recovery.

Karen returned to her parents' home in California and died on February 4 of the cardiac sequelae of her disease. She was eulogized in almost every significant publication, including the *Los Angeles Times* (Seiler, 1983), the *New York Times*, *People* magazine, the *Guardian* and various music publications like *Billboard* and on National Public Radio. Anorexia nervosa became widely recognized as a very serious disease!

On the 32nd anniversary of Carpenter's death, reporter Jennifer Latson of *Time* magazine wrote "*How Karen Carpenter's Death Changed the Way We Talk about Anorexia*" (2015). Carpenter's sad biography probably attracted more interest in the disease than all the scientific papers published to that time. Bruch's books, Carpenter's demise and other stories of dire consequences of anorexia catalyzed interest in anorexia and research of this potentially fatal disease.

Today, many books exist on anorexia nervosa, as well as limitless personal accounts and memoirs. PubMed listed more than 18,046 articles in February 2022, increasing slightly over past years but still not matching the 566,364 citations to articles on depression, for example. One study noted that articles on eating disorders were published less often than others in prominent medical and psychiatric journals; articles on eating disorders appeared largely in specialty journals (Frost et al., 2003).

References

Arcelus, J., Mitchell, A.J., Wales, J., & Nielsen, S. (2011). Mortality rates in patients with anorexia nervosa and other eating disorders. A meta-analysis of 36 studies. *Archives of General Psychiatry*, 68(7), 724–731.

Blumberg, J.J. (1982). Chlorotic girls, 1870-1920: a historical perspective on female adolescence. *Child Development*, 53(6), 1468–1477.

Bruch, H. (1973). *Eating Disorders: Obesity, Anorexia and the Person Within.* New York: Basic Books.

Bruch, H. (1978). *The Golden Cage: The Enigma of Anorexia Nervosa.* London: Open Books.

Crisp, A.H. (1968). Primary anorexia nervosa. *Gut*, 9(4), 370–372.

Dunbar, H.F. (1935). *Emotions and Bodily Changes: A Survey of Literature on Psychosomatic Interrelationships 1910-1933*. New York: Columbia University Press.

Eckert, E.D., Goldberg, S.C., Halmi, K.A., Casper, R.C., & Davis, J.M. (1979). Behavior therapy in anorexia nervosa. *British Journal of Psychiatry*, 134, 55–59.

Engel, G. (1980). The clinical application of the biopsychosocial model. *American Journal of Psychiatry*, 137(5), 535–544.

Frazier, S.H. (1963). Everything on anorexia. "Anorexia Nervosa Held to be Medical Crisis". *Medical Tribune*, November 18.

Frazier, S.H. (1970). Anorexia nervosa, *Hospital Medicine*, January, pp. 60–69.

Frost, S., Murphy, R., Webster, P., & Schmidt, U. (2003). Are top journals biased against eating disorders topics? *American Journal of Psychiatry*, 160(2), 363–369.

Gull, W.W. (1874). Anorexia nervosa (apepsia hysterica, anorexia hysterica). *Transactions of the Clinical Society of London*, 7, 221–228.

Halmi, K.A., Powers, P., & Cunningham, S. (1975). Treatment of anorexia nervosa with behavior modification. *Archives of General Psychiatry*, 32, 93–96.

Kaufman, M.R., & Heiman, M. (Eds.) (1964). *Evolution of Psychosomatic Concepts: Anorexia Nervosa: A Paradigm*. New York: International Universities Press, Inc.

Kluck, A.S., Garos, S., & Shaw, L. (2018). Sexual functioning and disordered eating: a new perspective. *Bulletin of the Menninger Clinic*, 82(1), 71–91.

Lasègue, C. (1873). On hysterical anorexia (*De l'Anorexie Hysterique*). *Medical Times and Gazette*, 2, 265–266, 367–369.

Latson, J. (2015). Karen Anne Carpenter. *Time Magazine*, February 4.

Lief, A. (1948). *The Commonsense Psychiatry of Dr. Adolf Meyer*. New York: McGraw-Hill.

Lipsitt, D.R. (1989). Anorexia nervosa, Felix Deutsch, and the associative anamnesis: a psychosomatic kaleidoscope, *Psychosomatic Medicine*, 51, 597–601.

Loudon, I.S. (1980). Chlorosis, anaemia, and anorexia nervosa. *British Medical Journal*, 281, 20–27.

Loudon, I.S. (1984). The diseases called chlorosis. *Psychological Medicine Journal*, 4(1), 27–36.

Morton, R. (1689). *Phthisiologia, or a Treatise of Consumption*. London: S. Smith & B. Walford.

Raciborski, A. (1865). *De l'amenorr par causes psychiques. Archives de Medicinehee*, 1, 521. Quoted in M.R. Kaufman & M. Heiman (1964) *Evolution of Psychosomatic Concepts: Anorexia Nervosa: A Paradigm*. New York: International Universities Press, Inc.

Ryle, J.A. (1936). Anorexia nervosa. *Lancet*, 2, 893–899.

Sayers, J. (1988). Anorexia, psychoanalysis and feminism: fantasy and reality. *Journal of Adolescence*, 11(4), 361–371.

Seiler, M. (1983). Karen Carpenter, half of soft-rock duo, dead at 32. *Los Angeles Times*, February 4, p. 2.

Shorter, E. (1992). *From Paralysis to Fatigue: A History of Psychosomatic Illness in the Modern Era*. New York: The Free Press.

Theriot, N.M. (1988). Psychosomatic illness in history: the "green sickness" among nineteenth century adolescent girls. *Journal of Psychohistory*, 15(4), 461–480.

Vigersky, R. (Ed.) (1977). *Anorexia Nervosa*. New York: Raven Press.

von Bertalanffy, L. (1968). *General Systems Theory: Foundations, Development, Applications*. New York: George Braziller.

Waller, J.V., Kaufman, M.R., & Deutsch, F. (1940). Anorexia nervosa: a psychosomatic entity. *Psychosomatic Medicine*, 2, 3–16.

3 The Patient, Her Mother, and Her Doctors

A psychobiological history constructed from extant notes and my knowledge of her will provide a useful matrix within which to view Ms. B's illness, one of the first cases of anorexia nervosa reported in the 20th century.

The Patient, Ms. B

On August 22, 1919, a baby girl was the first child born to its Russian immigrant parents. They lived in a small house in a relatively impoverished section of Boston where father worked as a tailor and mother as a homemaker. Mother, eager to assimilate in her new country, changed her proper name from Russian to American. The mother would later describe their home life as "normal" in the early days but intolerable by the time her daughter reached puberty. Copious notes exist but unfortunately do not include information about nursing behavior or other early infant–mother interaction.

Ms. B was said to have stuttered from the age of 5, not lasting into adolescence. As a young girl, she was considered attractive, intelligent, active and interested in life. She had friends and was especially attractive to young boys. In 1936, she graduated high school with honors at age 17. Her teachers liked her and encouraged her to apply to college. Her parents, however, nullified this option and urged her instead to find work. Employed briefly as a store clerk and office worker, she never afterward sought formal education or employment. She attended a camp run by a Massachusetts General Hospital (MGH) physician for two seasons in 1936–1938 at ages 17 and 18. At 19–20, she was brought by mother to Boston's Beth Israel Hospital (BIH) medical clinic because of a question of hyperthyroidism and weight loss from 138 to 87. Her records indicate that anorexia nervosa was first diagnosed at that time, October 8, 1938, and the next year she was seen in both psychiatry and endocrine clinics.

A first psychiatric hospital admission to Boston State Hospital (BSH) for a "washing compulsion" was recorded April 23, 1940 at age 21. Soon after (November–December, 1941), she was treated about one month at Boston

DOI: 10.4324/9781003208693-3

Psychopathic Hospital (BPH) (later renamed Massachusetts Mental Health Center, or MMHC). As an outpatient in March 1941, she was seen briefly by a renowned Boston psychoanalyst (no records available).

By 1944, at age 25, after much conflict and parental argument, she married an "older man." Her romantic interests were in a much younger man, but she felt "pushed" by parents, especially mother, to choose otherwise. (Romantic interest, marriage and divorce are topics of intense focus in all interview material.)

By the first month of 1946, at age 27, she was hospitalized at MMHC (January 8, 1946) for almost a year, then transferred by Dr. Robert Moss to Hartford's Institute for Living for 5 weeks. Mother, however, withdrew her against medical advice because "it was too expensive." (As long ago as 1895, Stephens [1895] noted exacerbation of the anorexic patient's illness with mothers' frequent visits to their hospitalized daughters.)

By November, 1949, Ms. B divorced. Again, she was admitted for less than one month to BSH after threatening mother with a knife. There followed a brief visit to BIH's outpatient psychiatry clinic, where she was seen by Dr. S, and within 3 months she was back at MMHC continuing with Dr. S. During this time, psychological testing recorded an IQ of 122, a verbal IQ of 181, and conflictual presence around aggression with a tendency to denigrate herself. In the patient's responses to imagery cards, she held that "outside forces push you around," that "men kill you in sex," that "to be a woman is to be helpless," and that "femininity is valueless." The psychologist proposed the diagnosis of "mixed neurosis," adding that although she "tests reality well grossly, she lives in fantasy," that she is "functionally but not structurally, psychotic," nevertheless, "not schizophrenic."

In 1951, when she was 31, a man, possibly her divorced husband, committed suicide. She became depressed and withdrawn, and her phobic and obsessive-compulsive behavior worsened. A breast biopsy, for unspecified reasons, performed in 1954 at New England Medical Center, was followed by symptoms of increased fatigue, decreased energy and greater indecisiveness. Records of biopsy results are not available.

At age 37, in 1956, she was treated at Worcester State Hospital, perhaps for late post-surgical depression, with 24 electroconvulsive therapy (ECT) treatments. Seen in the BIH Emergency Ward that same year, she was medically hospitalized with acute thrombophlebitis; major complaints besides leg pain were abdominal pain, constipation, weight loss and amenorrhea. Follow-up visits were arranged in both endocrine and medical clinics for treatment and care of swollen legs, constipation, and abdominal pain. In psychiatric consultation with Dr. T, she was placed on disability and referred to Jewish Family and Children's Service to be followed by a social worker.

In June, 1960, at age 41, Ms. B was admitted to BIH for evaluation of "various somatic complaints" thought possibly related to an endocrinological disorder. Her ward physician requested a repeat psychiatric consultation, feeling that there was insufficient assessment of this aspect of her illness. Ward physicians described her as "seemingly well-adjusted, well-liked and even helpful on the ward, although bedridden and isolated at home." During hospitalization, though active, she complained of "no energy." She had a normal period and weight was 135. Again, hypothyroidism was *treated* with thyroid extract in October 1960. Because she appeared alert and likeable, medical opinion suggested that "perhaps further help (presumably psychiatric) should be offered her at this time." The social worker made note of a disturbing relationship at home with mother, who made veiled threats of suicide if her daughter was to be returned home.

Dr. Meiss of the Psychiatric Service at BIH saw the patient in consultation and recorded "the patient had been thoroughly evaluated (medically) and found to be in good physical health." An extensive evaluation by Dr. Meiss described the patient as "severely psychiatrically disturbed since her middle teens when she was seen by Dr. [Felix] Deutsch who made a diagnosis of anorexia nervosa." According to Dr. Meiss's history, the patient "had seen at least 5 psychiatrists and various social workers and in each instance has terminated the relationship." Psychiatric hospitalization was recorded on two occasions while she resided at home with mother and father. Employment was brief and discontinuous, and she was increasingly withdrawn and isolated. Social contacts were virtually nonexistent, and complaints of "bodily aches and pains, swelling and redness of legs and feet" continued.

Comparing data from the patient herself with that obtained in consultation 2 years previously, Dr. Meiss ascertained that there was "no appreciable change in mental status or behavior," or "shift in her relationship with parents." Dr. Meiss's note described the patient as "a pleasant-looking woman who appears much younger than her stated age and has a childish and clinging quality." The patient

> spoke eagerly, clearly happy to be interviewed. Tears welled up with little provocation with crying seemingly unrelated to any obvious deep depression or particular mental content. The patient related her entire life as one in which she had been mistreated and the victim of others and circumstances.

Throughout Dr. Meiss's interview, the patient "was extremely bland, without obvious disturbance of affect or thought processes." Though "presently well-oriented, she was extremely vague about past dates and events. Regarding future plans, none were in evidence." Much of Ms. B's extensive vocalizing focused on topics known from previous interviews: good student, always on honor roll; encouraged by teachers to go to college but obstructed by parents, insisting she go to work; being ignored and told lies about by parents; mistreated because she was a girl and "a girl is nothing to them"; in love in her mid-teens with "a man she wanted to marry but mother broke up the relationship"; "no confidence in myself, feel like a child"; "stopped seeing friends because of emotional problems"; "sorry that my parents hate me so; she (mother) used to beat me and tear me to pieces." Her marriage was "only a crutch," another way to "get away from home."

Extremely vague on this occasion about her psychiatric history, she thought that psychiatrists were more interested in her mother than in her. She did recall that mother had first taken her in late 1930s to psychiatric clinic when she had lost a great deal of weight. That was the time she started washing her hands excessively because she "felt dirty after a man at work had made sexual advances" toward her.

Acknowledging to Dr. Meiss that she failed to follow through with psychiatrist or social worker on last hospitalization, she "explained" that "doctors and social workers couldn't do everything for me, that I have to help myself." Dr. Meiss, however, experienced little genuine sense of responsibility in the patient's remark. The social worker added mother's complaint that her daughter stayed up all night, insisting that food be brought to her at odd hours, and that she was argumentative, sometimes even violent, "probably out of control of herself."

Summing up her contact with Ms. B, Dr. Meiss wrote that

> although she has been previously diagnosed with anorexia nervosa and compulsion neurosis, presently the symptoms (of those conditions) are not present, and my impression is of an oral narcissistic character disorder. Her chronicity and severity totally incapacitate her and would raise the question of whether she might have been actively psychotic in the past.

Recommendations by Dr. Meiss included, once again, referral to a social worker at Jewish Family and Children's Service. Dr. Meiss added that

> prognosis is extremely poor, and that the patient can only be helped in terms of stabilizing her and preventing further deterioration. There is no indication that the patient is amenable to psychotherapy or that she wants to separate from her long, hostile-dependent relationship with her mother.

About one month later, on July 11, 1960, Dr. Meiss was asked to see the patient again during hospitalization, more to interview the patient's mother and to assist the social worker in managing the latter. A short note about Ms. B said "no change from recent consultation (of June 14)."

Sexual history, obtained later, suggested that Ms. B did not become aware of genital sexuality and pregnancy until age 12. However, she masturbated before and after that age and had also been aware of the births of her two brothers. She slept in the same bed with older brother from age 6 to 8. They ate in bed and engaged in sexual play. She thought that kissing was responsible for pregnancy but believed that babies were born only in marriage. Thinking that sex was dirty and that masturbation caused abnormalities, purification rituals and signs of compulsive eating began around age 12 as she tried to discontinue masturbation. At age 16, she was attracted to a boy she said was "impulsive and sexually attractive." She said that was when she began overeating and then broke up with him in less than a year.

On her way home one day, a boy exposed himself to her and demanded intercourse, causing her to be "upset." On another occasion, she was "picked up by two Italian boys who tried to attack her," but she fled. Once during the short time she worked (not known when), "an old man lifted my skirt." A note in her medical record states that "mother paid fifteen dollars to have her 'opened up,' but no further details exist."

By July 23, 1960, at age 41, Ms. B was seen again in the BIH Emergency Ward and transferred to BSH, from which she was promptly withdrawn by mother. In a repeat episode of an Emergency Ward admission at BIH, on October 11, 1961, I met the patient for the first time (see "First Encounter").

In 1968, when Ms. B's mother died at age 69, Ms. B was 49. Ms. B entered a nursing home and, after 16 years in two different homes, moved with a nursing home companion to a communal housing apartment, where she lived until her death. Events toward the end of her life are vague. Hospital visits had diminished and records are incomplete. It was rumored that she had applied to a day program in the face of questionable abuse at home, but further records are unavailable.

Additional details of Ms. B's history are revealed in the several interviews replicated here.

The Mother, Mrs. B (Description from Clinical Notes and Personal Encounters)

Ms. B repeatedly described her mother as a difficult person, with whom she had many arguments, "fights" and conflicts. She frequently bemoaned the fact that "I don't understand why she hates me so."

In a review of 16 anorexia cases, Cobb (1950, p. 179) states, "in every one of our cases, there were badly disturbed parental relations, usually with a scolding and overbearing mother."

My own first knowledge of the patient's mother (Mrs. B) derives from medical records of 1954, about 15 years after her daughter's diagnosis of anorexia, a time when mother was seeking care and treatment for her own maladies. During a medical visit when she complained of pain in her legs and breasts, her doctor observed "agitation" and seemed dismissively to advise "a brassiere with more uplift" and referred her to psychiatry.

A psychiatrist consultant (Dr. Kanter) interviewed her before a group of medical students (for instructional purposes). The interview elicited personal psychological and medical history and paid considerable attention to relationship with her daughter.

Mrs. B immigrated from Russia to the United States at age 15, after father died when she was 9 (no comment made about her mother). She married a man who was a "boyfriend" of her brother, saying she never loved him but needed him because "he made a living." She described having gone to visit him in the Army in 1918 and "he didn't want to see me." Husband was characterized as a soldier injured in the war and easily aggravated, yelling at and beating the daughter and "yelling at me." "We've never gotten along well." She said he avoided eating when he was angry.

Mrs. B's first pregnancy was in 1919. She had wondered whether she was able to become pregnant but "wanted a baby because my sister had one." Describing the close relationship with her daughter, she said they slept together during daughter's early years and adolescence. Mother said the little girl stuttered from the age 5 but outgrew it. "She teased others and didn't like to be told what to do, and never kept her promises."

This first child was portrayed as a "clean, compulsive girl, who could never keep appointments, just like me, always late." Though "always attractive to boys and very attractive to men," according to mother, "when they called for her, she ran out the back door to be with a girlfriend." Mother said that daughter always blamed her for difficulties with boys.

Mother admitted she would like to beat her and complained she made sacrifices for her by washing her clothes and doing other tasks. According to mother, her daughter married a man she didn't love; he later hanged himself. Describing this sequence of events, Mrs. B laughed and said "I want to kill my husband too."

The story that a doctor had once told Ms. B that her mother hated her because she was a girl was angrily denied by mother. As for her own medical care, she said "doctors can either help or kill. Doctors make me crazy." "I don't know why I am here in the psychiatry department; I need to be given to." "I wouldn't mind seeing a social worker because one once helped my daughter go to summer camp." Her daughter was being seen at a hospital different from her mother's, had twice been in the local psychiatric hospital, and was now being seen in outpatient clinic.

Dr. Kanter's post-conference note indicated "This patient is indeed a very disturbed woman." Further, he recorded that "her problems center around her own personality, her husband and her daughter." Her medical history at the time listed repeat operative procedures, dilation and curettage (D&C), excision of vaginal mucosa and repair of cystocele and rectocele. Attention to her own "female" problems was in marked evidence.

No data was obtained about Mrs. B's relation to her own mother, a potentially useful source of information regarding the influence of trans-generational transmission of attachment abnormalities (Ward, Ramsay & Treasure, 2000) from mothers to daughters. Noteworthy is the fact that Mrs. B came to this country around her own puberty or early post-puberty years and in all likelihood was not successful in boy–girl relationships, marrying only as "a convenience." No further information was obtained about her siblings, apparently a brother and sister.

The psychiatrist's concluding summary stated

> This 56-year-old woman is a terribly hostile, orally demanding woman whose basic attachment seems to be a sadomasochistic one with her daughter. A loveless relationship with her husband is easily acknowledged together with her tolerance of him ('to whatever degree she can be tolerant') based on his making a living. There are overt death wishes to both husband and daughter. It is felt that this patient is essentially untreatable and is not motivated to treatment, but toward a demanding hostile dependency. No further contact.

Nonetheless, she was referred to the Social Service Department because of her "agitation" where an extensive recap of her medical history was recorded. She had first been admitted to BIH on January 28, 1948 for "dropped womb." (Her daughter was 28 at the time.) The procedures of repair of cystocele and rectocele, D&C, anterior and posterior colporrhaphy and cervical amputation were again noted. In a second medical admission 7 ½ months later, she complained of "vaginal discomfort." It was the doctor's impression that she was "suffering from an anxiety neurosis." She was discharged in four days but readmitted almost one year later with a question of "menopausal bleeding." She described irregular menses for many months and recent staining and hot flashes. A sigmoidoscopy was inexplicably performed, and she was discharged 5 days later.

In an earlier social work contact, at the time of her first medical admission in February 1948, Mrs. B requested "help in making plans for daughter's care." She was described as "having personality problems and evidence of mental disturbance." The record indicates that daughter "had been treated by many psychiatrists and hospitalized a number of times." Mother "stated that her daughter's troubles began about 10 years previously (1938) when the man she was engaged to tried to attack her (not clear from patient interviews), causing her to feel dirty and needing to wash herself constantly." Mother complained that daughter "made me do everything for her." Social worker entries say "all the doctors she went to told mother to let daughter live by self, but daughter would stay away for a while and then come home to sleep with her mother." Mrs. B said she wanted help from social service to "get her daughter out of the house." Discussion ensued about having the daughter assessed at MMHC for advisability of a lobectomy! This was not pursued. The "case was closed" in April of 1948 but reopened in social service 3 years later with mother again complaining of daughter being at home, asking social worker to assist in removing her from the home. A suggestion that Mrs. B herself see a psychiatrist elicited the response that "a psychiatrist could not help her and she just wanted help to make plans to send her daughter away."

Over the years, Mrs. B was seen by sequential social workers, most of whom confirmed the psychiatrists' and previous social workers' assessments that she was "not treatable." She was often late, just as she described herself. In my own time following her daughter, the mother frequently interfered with daughter's appointments, often countermanded recommendations, first encouraging daughter's hospitalization and then signing her out against medical advice. Many letters and phone calls to me or my secretaries followed, importuning all who would listen to complaints about her daughter or herself. On one occasion, very shortly after I had seen Ms. B for the first time, her mother called my office leaving word that she wanted to talk with me but that I shouldn't call her "because my very sick daughter might be around." She asked that I write her a letter giving a time when she could come talk with me. This seemed the beginning of a very intense effort to competitively engage me, ostensibly to provide important information (complaints) about her daughter.

I quote from one typewritten letter to me, January 7, 1963 (about 2 years after my first encounter with Ms. B):

> Dear Dr. Lipsitt:
>
> I am the unhappy mother of your patient and conditions at home are so bad that I am forced to write to you. I know no where (sic) to turn and because I need help for [my daughter's] behalf, I am writing to you about her condition.
>
> To begin with [my daughter] goes to sleep only once in every four nights; she takes no solid food and I am safe in saying that since she came home from the Recuperative Center, she has only once taken food that was solid. She only drinks—pepsi-cola or orange juice.
>
> [She] is afraid to stay in the house, afraid to go to bed. But on the fourth night, since her legs are so badly swollen, and she can't stand on her feet, she is forced to go to bed. Before she goes to bed, she shakes herself, starts chocking (sic), afraid that she will die, and neither will she allow me to go to bed.
>
> I must tell you about "bundles." Not alone she wraps her own items in paper wrappers, but now she also wraps my own underwear, my towels; she even wraps my drawers and wraps my belongings. So then she becomes very nervous, because she can't find an item she has already wrapped—because all bundles look alike to her. She even wraps paper with paper. Then she places all these bundles on her bed, so the result is she has no place to sleep. This has to really be seen to believe just what a sight it is.

> The only good point about her is her ability to talk well. Her medical condition is far from well. Her feet are swollen, so that she could hardly walk. [She] bleeds both from the rectum as well as the vagina—off and on.
>
> I know you have recommended that [she] come in to the EW and then for observation—but how can she come when she never gets dressed, never leaves the house, and always says that she is "dirty" and needs a bath badly, but she never has time to take a bath, according to her way of living.
>
> [She] finds excuses for not doing things, for not going to the [hospital], for not getting dressed, and so forth. It is next to impossible to stand from her, and I am at the end of my rope. Both my husband and myself are sick from her actions and do not know where to turn. Is it possible to send a Doctor from the [hospital] or elsewhere, for him to "bring" her to the hospital? Otherwise, she will never go herself. Both my husband and I want to live—live for our other children and grandchildren, but how can we with her in our house, complaining all the time, how sick she is and groaning to us that she is going to die, YET she does nothing about it.
>
> I would like to add this: [my daughter] tells me, that if she did not live in the house, she would go to sleep every night. The same with food—she eats like a normal person everywhere, except in my house.
>
> I could go on and on, without end.
>
> If it is possible for you to send a doctor to my house, or for you to recommend to me the name of a doctor whom I should contact for the purpose of taking [her] to the [hospital], I would be more than willing to pay this doctor his regular fee. I do not want this doctor to come to my house and not get paid for his visit.
>
> If you would like to see me after you have read this letter, my phone number is [xxx-xxxx].
>
> Thank you for your interest in *my* (my italics) case.
>
> Very truly yours,
>
> Mrs. B

In one of her interviews, Ms. B said "My mother says I'm hopeless and I try to show her I'm just what she says I am."

Interestingly relevant to the case of Ms. B, most reported psychoanalytic cases mention prominence of mother in fostering and maintaining the illness. Virtually every clinical case report noted the sentinel role of the mother in etiology or endurance of the disease. Waller, Kaufman and Deutsch (Kaufman & Heiman, 1964, p. 259) state: "It seems that in the patients who develop anorexia nervosa the mother relationship plays a rather specific and significant role." This is indisputable in the case of Ms. B. Undoubtedly, this verity stimulated the expansion of family therapy (see the "Ascendance of Family Therapy" section in Chapter 6).

Charcot, one of Freud's early teachers, quotes: "Experience shows repeatedly, though it is not always easy to understand the reason, that it is the mothers whose influence is so deleterious, who will hear no argument, and will only yield in general to the last extremity" (Kaufman & Heiman, 1964, p. 163).

Sir William W. Gull, in one of the earliest suggestions of the effect of the family on the patient, "paid special attention to the intrafamily relationship, the effect of the family on the patient and the reverse" (Kaufman & Heiman, 1964, p. 143). The German physician, Weizsacker, studied dreams of patients with anorexia (Weizsacker, 1937) and found that they most often included reference to mothers (p. 166).

The concept of the etiologic role of the schizophrenogenic mother of schizophrenia has long been abandoned in psychiatric research and literature. Nonetheless, given the early and close relation from birth of children to their mothers, it is not totally unreasonable to attempt to understand any dysfunction of the developmental process in that aspect of the relationship. In anorexia nervosa, no writer has suggested an "anorexogenic" mother–daughter relationship, but all reports of the disease, as indicated, since Gull and Lasègue refer to the strong role that mothers have in how they respond to their anorexic daughters and vice versa.

The Patient's Physicians

Dr. John Waller

Although Dr. Waller is lead author of a seminal paper about Ms. B, little biographical data is available. It is assumed that he was a resident-in-training from the nature of his interview and involvement of "mentors" like Drs. Felix Deutsch and M. Ralph Kaufman. A search reveals no other publications by him. Attribution of institutional sources of the paper, co-authored with Kaufman and Deutsch, lists Medical Research Laboratory and Psychiatric Clinic of Boston's BIH and the Department of Medicine of Harvard Medical School; individual affiliations of authors are not listed.

Dr. Felix Deutsch

Dr. Deutsch was born in Vienna in 1885, attended medical school there, graduated at age 25 and practiced first as an internist before becoming a psychoanalyst, during which time (1922–1923) he had been Freud's personal internist. He had been chair of medicine at University of Vienna as well as at a neighboring hospital before entering training as a psychoanalyst. Dual interests in medicine and psychoanalysis likely formed a latticework for pursuit of mind–body relationships and psychosomatic medicine as seen in the evolution of his unique style of interviewing patients, termed "associative anamnesis" (Deutsch, 1939) based partly on the psychoanalytic concept of free association. He is credited with having coined the expressions "psychosomatic medicine" and "psychosomatic unit" (Deutsch, 1959), the blending of both mental and physical aspects of a patient's illness (Deutsch, 1960). The interview of Ms. B in 1938 illustrates his technique (see Dr. Deutsch's interview with the patient in the "Dr. Deutsch's Encounter with Ms. B" section of Chapter 4).

Deutsch emigrated to the United States in 1935, hosted by Dr. Stanley Cobb, chairman of a newly formed general hospital psychiatric service at MGH. As an avid psychoanalyst, Deutsch became a founder and president of the Boston Psychoanalytic Society and Institute (BPSI) and faculty member of both BIH and MGH.

He spent almost his entire career in the Boston and Cambridge areas in psychoanalytic practice, consulting and teaching in several hospitals, one exception an invitation to be the first professor of psychosomatic medicine at University of Washington Medical School from 1939 to 1941.

Deutsch was described as a kind of *wunderkind* with interest and talent in art, music, composing and poetry, skills he brought into his psychoanalytic work with literary publications.

Eulogized by his colleague Dr. William F. Murphy (1964, p. 424) as "a kindly, sensitive man of dignified mien, a fascinating teacher, and, above all, a tireless and original thinker," he was highly esteemed by students, colleagues and others for his ideas and skill as a pioneer in psychosomatic medicine, including the application of medicine, psychoanalysis and psychiatry to the care and treatment of patients. His extensive work included seminal papers on the process of conversion by which emotional conflict was transformed and manifested as somatic presentation. He also wrote an important reassessment of Freud's Dora case (Deutsch, 1957).

In his brief interaction in 1938 with Waller's patient, Deutsch demonstrated (for students, trainees and staff) application of the technique of associative anamnesis. His brief interaction with Ms. B made a significant impression on her, for she vividly remembered him decades later. The case described here and published in 1940 (Waller, Kaufman & Deutsch, 1940) was first presented by Deutsch to a meeting of the American Psychoanalytic Association in Chicago in May 1938, to be published in the journal *Psychosomatic Medicine*. In spite of his commitment to psychoanalytic treatment, Deutsch cautioned

> in case the psychiatric interview has revealed that psychic factors play an important role in the symptomatology of the sickness, or else that the organic process which seems to be the core of the illness is only the partial expression of a neurosis, then *one has to decide whether a deep-digging psychotherapeutic method like psychoanalysis should be recommended* (my italics).
>
> (Deutsch, 1927 in Kaufman & Heiman, 1964, p. 52)

Dr. M. Ralph Kaufman

Dr. M. Ralph Kaufman's interest in anorexia as a psychosomatic paradigm probably germinated much before Waller's experience. Russian-born Kaufman received his medical degree from McGill University, psychiatric training at BPH (later MMHC) and psychoanalytic training at the Vienna Psychoanalytic Institute, analyzed by Dr. P.F. in 1929.

On return to Boston, Kaufman was a founding member of the Boston Psychoanalytic Institute and, like Deutsch, president (1937–1939), chairman of the Education Committee (1934–1942) and consulting psychiatrist at MGH. Volunteering for the Army in World War II, he returned to Boston to briefly hold the position of Chairman of the Department of Psychiatry at BIH before being recruited by Mount Sinai Hospital in New York to chair their department of psychiatry. His interest in anorexia nervosa never left him from his time at MGH, and in 1964 with co-author Marcel Heiman, he produced the seminal text *Evolution of Psychosomatic Concepts: Anorexia Nervosa: A Paradigm*. This essential volume contains the deliberations of the Mount Sinai Seminar Group [on Anorexia], chaired by Kaufman, as well as an edited compendium of basic papers (as of 1964) on anorexia nervosa, with commentary by Kaufman and Heiman. Contained therein is the paper by Waller, Kaufman & Deutsch, including a description of "our" patient, and the 1927 paper by Deutsch on *Psychoanalysis and Medicine*, where the expressions "psychosomatic medicine" and "psychosomatic unit" appear. Accompanying commentary by Kaufman asserts that "the feeding stimulus becomes the most important factor for the foundation of the ego structure" (Kaufman & Heiman, 1964, p. 48). This paper formed the groundwork for Deutsch's "associative anamnesis."

Dr. John Romano

As founding chairman of Rochester University School of Medicine and Dentistry's Department of Psychiatry, Dr. Romano was one of America's foremost psychiatric educators. During his early training years in 1938–1939, he received a Rockefeller Fellowship to study neurology at Boston City Hospital. From 1939 to 1941, he also received a fellowship to study psychoanalysis as a Sigmund Freud Fellow of BPSI. In the same years in Boston, he became acquainted with Dr. Milton Rosenbaum, in psychiatric training at MGH-McLean Hospital. They became close friends with mutual interests in psychiatry and psychosomatic medicine. Dr. Romano, as part of his training, was assigned Ms. B as a psychosomatic patient with anorexia, a case he later presented to a seminar at the Psychoanalytic Institute. His meticulous notes on both patient and her mother as well as seminar records are reflected in this monograph.

As mentioned in the preamble to this account, it was Dr. Rosenbaum who first alerted Dr. Romano to my 1989 paper, eliciting from him his copious typewritten notes from more than 50 years ago! The patient was interviewed by him briefly, perhaps for a two-hour interview, on May 14, 1941, another time in June, and presented to the seminar at BPSI on December 16, 1941 where the case was discussed by Drs. Helene Deutsch, her husband Felix, Erich Lindemann, Charles Brenner and Helen Tartakoff and other noted Boston psychoanalysts. Reference to the content of that seminar, especially comments of Dr. Helene Deutsch, were retrieved from archives and published by Dr. Paul Roazen (1981). (Extracts of that conference will be discussed in Dr. Romano's segment of the story of Ms. B.)

In 1942, Dr. Romano was recruited by the University of Cincinnati to head their psychiatry department, where he remained until moving to Rochester 3 years later to establish one of the country's most progressive clinical training and research psychiatry departments.

Dr. Robert M. Eisendrath

Dr. Eisendrath was a senior resident in psychiatry and psychoanalyst-in-training at the time he interviewed Ms. B during her hospitalization at BIH in 1961. His interview is reproduced in its entirety to demonstrate the enduring themes of earlier interviews. Dr. Eisendrath had been familiar with Dr. Felix Deutsch's 1938 account of Ms. B.

Dr. Don R. Lipsitt (Author)

Dr. Lipsitt was a senior psychiatric resident and psychoanalyst-in-training in the Department of Psychiatry of BIH, chaired by Dr. Grete Bibring, a Vienna-trained psychoanalyst, whose pioneering influence on application of psychoanalytic precepts to medical settings is richly explicated in her classic article in the *New England Journal of Medicine* in 1956. Drs. Eisendrath and Lipsitt were beneficiaries of Dr. Bibring's teaching and supervision. As consulting psychiatrist, Dr. Lipsitt first encountered the patient when he was summoned as a psychiatric consultant to the Emergency Ward of BIH on October 11, 1961 (curiously, a near anniversary of the date of her diagnosis on October 8, 1938), the experience and sequelae that form this account of the patient's 60-plus-year course of illness.

Further Reading

Bruch, H. (1973). *Eating Disorders: Obesity, Anorexia and the Person Within.* New York: Basic Books.

Bruch, H. (1978). *The Golden Cage: The Enigma of Anorexia Nervosa.* New York: Vintage Books.

Gull, W.W. (1873). (Translated from *Archives Generales de Medicine*, April, 1873, p. 143 in Kaufman & Heimen). *Evolution of Psychosomatic Concepts: Anorexia Nervosa: A Paradigm.* New York: International Universities Press, 1964.

Lasègue, C. (1873). On hysterical anorexia (*De l'Anorexie Hysterique*). *Medical Times and Gazette*, 2, 265–266, 367–369.

Phipps Psychiatric Clinic. (1966). *Learning about the patient's attitudes. Teaching guide for psychiatry residents (after Adolf Meyer). Unsigned.* Baltimore, MD: Johns Hopkins University. August 18, 1966, pp. 2–32.

Vigersky, R. (Ed.) (1977). *Anorexia Nervosa*. New York: Raven Press.

White, B.V. (1984). *Stanley Cobb: A Builder of the Modern Neurosciences*. Charlottesville: University of Virginia Press.

References

Charcot, J.M. (1889). *Diseases of the Nervous System*. London: New Sydenham Society. In M.R. Kaufman & M. Heiman (Eds.) (1964) *Evolution of Psychosomatic Concepts: Anorexia Nervosa: A Paradigm*. New York: International Universities Press, pp. 60–163.

Cobb, S., & Reid, J.R. (1950). *Emotions and Clinical Medicine*. New York: W.W. Norton & Co.

Deutsch, F. (1927). Psychoanalysis and internal medicine. In M.R. Kaufman & M. Heiman (Eds.) (1964) *Evolution of Psychosomatic Concepts: Anorexia Nervosa: A Paradigm*. New York: International Universities Press, pp. 47–55.

Deutsch, F. (1939). The associative anamnesis. *Psychoanalytic Quarterly*, 8, 354–381.

Deutsch, F. (1957). A footnote to Freud's "Fragment of an analysis of a case of hysteria". *Psychoanalytic Quarterly*, 26(2), 159–167.

Deutsch, F. (1959). Correlations of verbal and nonverbal communication in interviews elicited by the associative anamnesis. *Psychosomatic Medicine*, 21(2), 123–130.

Deutsch, F. (1960). Entering the mind through the sensory gateways in associative anamnesis. *Psychosomatic Medicine*, 27(6), 466–480.

Kaufman, M.R., & Heiman, M. (Eds.) (1964). *Psychosomatic Medicine, Evolution of Psychosomatic Concepts: Anorexia Nervosa: A Paradigm*. New York: International Universities Press, Inc.

Murphy, W.F. (1964). Felix Deutsch 1884-1964. *The Psychoanalytic Quarterly*, 33(3), 424–426.

Roazen, P. (1981). Anorexia nervosa: Helene Deutsch, M.D. *Bulletin of the Menninger Clinic*, 45(6), 499–501.

Stephens, I.E.W. (1895). Case of anorexia nervosa: necropsy. *Lancet*, 1, 31–32.

Waller, J.V., Kaufman, M.R., & Deutsch, F. (1940). Anorexia nervosa: a psychosomatic entity. *Psychosomatic Medicine*, 2, 3–16.

Ward, A., Ramsay, R., & Treasure, J. (2000). Attachment research in eating disorders. *British. Journal of Medical Psychology*, 73, 35–51.

Weizsacker, V.V. (1937). Dreams in so-called endogenic *magersucht* (anorexia). In M.R. Kaufman & M. Heiman (Eds.) (1964) *Evolution of Psychosomatic Concepts: Anorexia Nervosa: A Paradigm*. New York: International Universities Press, pp. 166, 181.

4 Interview Sequence

> The study of developmental processes represents one of the cornerstones in efforts to understand human psychic functioning. An appreciation of the movement from the immature to the mature, from the less complex to the highly complicated, from reflexive neonatal patterns to multi-determined symbolic behavior, from the biological to the psychological, and from external forces to internal structure is fundamental to formulating a general psychology of man as well as to the delineation of those processes that are at the root of neurogenesis.
>
> – N. Fischer, 1989, p. 41

Early Encounters

In the early 1900s, when Dr. Adolf Meyer espoused a psychobiological approach to understanding patients in their entirety, both psyche and soma, he stressed the importance of the art of history-taking in achieving that objective (Phipps Psychiatric Clinic, 1966). He taught his students the importance of a patient's attitudes and personality throughout developmental stages, "how to deal with the psychobiological unit—the person—in action." "Common examples of such combinations of behavioral and visceral disorders associated with anxiety are found in fastidiousness toward food, easy disgustibility, dizziness and even amenorrhea, as illustrated in anorexia nervosa" (Phipps Psychiatric Clinic, 1966, p. 12). The interviews reproduced here demonstrate that principle as well as Fischer's "delineation of those processes that are at the root of [the patient's] neurogenesis" (see Fischer, 1989).

Although Ms. B had apparently been seen by several psychiatrists over time, records exist only from the following: John V. Waller, M.D., M. Ralph Kaufman, M.D., Felix Deutsch, M.D., John Romano, M.D., Ellie Meiss, M.D., Stanley Kanter, M.D., Robert Eisendrath, M.D. and Don R. Lipsitt, M.D.

DOI: 10.4324/9781003208693-4

The first extant notation about Ms. B was made by psychiatric trainee John Waller at the Massachusetts General Hospital (MGH) on October 24, 1938. He saw patient and mother sequentially. Ms. B had been brought by her mother and admitted to Beth Israel Hospital (BIH) "with extreme progressive loss of weight" at least two weeks prior to Waller's first interview. With inpatient refeeding and support, she gained sufficient weight to be discharged in a few days and then was followed at MGH by Dr. Waller.

Perhaps the MGH was the ideal setting for Ms. B. The chairman of the Psychiatric Department was Dr. Stanley Cobb (1950), who, with support and encouragement from the Rockefeller Foundation, had been lured away from Boston City Hospital by Dr. Alan Gregg (Lipsitt, 2020), medical director of the Foundation, to establish one of the first psychiatric departments in a general hospital in the United States (Lipsitt, 2017).

Cobb was an exemplary physician to start a psychiatry service in a general hospital. He was a scientist, neuropathologist, neurologist, physiologist and psychiatrist who had studied at the Johns Hopkins School of Medicine. He was esteemed as innovative and receptive to new ideas, believing that no distinction was to be made between organic and mental illnesses.

At a time when psychoanalysis was establishing itself as a major contributor to psychiatric knowledge, Cobb expressed great interest in blending it into training at MGH, to foster understanding of the complexities of mind–body relations in psychosomatic illness. Though not a psychoanalyst himself, he had been analyzed and urged all his staff to undertake such treatment.

As previously mentioned, he welcomed psychoanalyst emigres from Nazi Germany and Austria in the early 1930s. These included Drs. Helene and Felix Deutsch, Grete and Edward Bibring, Lucie Jessner and Jenny and Robert Waelder, all of whom became members of Boston's psychoanalytic community and its Psychoanalytic Institute.

Cobb had hosted Carl Jung in 1936 on the occasion of the latter's conferred honorary degree at Harvard. And with James Jackson Putnam's admiration for Freud's ideas, Cobb was also instrumental in establishing psychoanalysis as a major discipline in the United States.

The 1930s also saw the heyday of psychosomatic medicine with the publication of the first journal of that movement in 1939 by Dr. Flanders Dunbar and the founding of the American Psychosomatic Society (*Psychosomatic Medicine*) in 1942. Articles in the journal were largely by psychoanalysts who saw the fruitful merging of psychoanalytic and psychosomatic trends in medicine. An important early paper on anorexia nervosa by Dr. L. Rahman and associates was published in the first volume of *Psychosomatic Medicine* in 1939 (Rahman, Richardson & Ripley, 1939).

An archival remembrance of Cobb (White, 1984, pp. 166, 181) states "At one conference attended by Cobb in about 1936, a patient with anorexia nervosa was presented and Cobb in his summary concluded that anorexia nervosa was a disease in its own right, not a manifestation of schizophrenia."

In this stimulating psychoanalytic/psychosomatic milieu, Ms. B's care was transferred from BIH to MGH, to be followed by Dr. Waller from October 1938 to March 1939, ending with disappointing results, then transferred to MGH staff member Dr. Lucie Jessner, a senior psychoanalyst, with the notation by Waller that "I am apparently not able to get to the basis of this neurosis and, on Dr. Kaufman's advice, will attempt to turn the patient over to Dr. Jessner Monday morning." Dr. Waller, at the end of his contact with Ms. B, atypically appended a countertransferential personal note in the chart about the patient's undesirability. (No further notes are available regarding this transfer.)

Apparently, the case of Ms. B had generated great interest at MGH since "heavy hitters" Drs. M. Ralph Kaufman and Felix Deutsch had been invited to consult. Dr. Kaufman interviewed Ms. B on January 23, 1939. Waller's notes of Kaufman's assessment disclose that "her problem at present was the terrific conflict with her mother" and that her "mother would never change." Kaufman commented that "patient does not remember any jealousy of her mother for her father's affection" and "during childhood, when she was afraid to go to bed, she slept with her parents, sleeping between them, the usual purpose being to keep them apart." His formulation stated that

> her mother has definitely been trying to live her own life over through her daughter in that she always says, 'if you could eat more, it would be better for <u>us</u>, that this boyfriend is good for <u>us</u> and that one is bad for <u>us</u>.'

In the anticipated advent of separation or loss of the daughter through death, Kaufman predicted that "her mother would probably mourn a month or less." "[But] the daughter on the other hand, would mourn for months of tears if her mother died." The patient "had a strong feeling of unity with the mother and at other times hated her" and "by this and her other actions, was punishing the mother," engendering guilt through which "her present habits were of such a nature that they would injure the mother as well as herself." Kaufman speculated that, with this behavior, "she would revert to childhood and have some authority at home to direct herself and her parents in relation to one another." In a direct comment to patient, he explained that neither she nor her mother would change without "further elucidation and bringing out the basic reasons for resentment against the mother [in order that] she could understand it and be able to handle it in a natural way." This assessment proved prescient without ever being achieved!

Dr. Waller's Notes

Because Dr. Waller's interview is seminal to all reports on this patient, examples of his earliest and latest clinical notes from October 24, 1938 to March 6, 1939 are reproduced as written by him while notes from November 30, 1938 to February 14, 1939 are excerpted and summarized. (Photographs of Dr. Waller's typewritten notes appear in Figures 4.1–4.6.)

O. P. D. 23

NAME [redacted] NO. 52687

October 24, 1938
Mother accompanies patient this morning; patient seen first.

There is no complaint at present; patient says she is fine.

History of case: Pt. was admitted to the Beth Israel Hospital about two weeks ago with extreme, progressive loss of weight. While in the hospital she gained about six pounds and was discharged after several days. Pt. has always quarreled violently with her mother; she can remember her mother interfering in her activities from earliest childhood. She states that mother is very good to her, in fact, that she has spoiled her, but still she objects very violently to her mother's attentions and has outbursts of temper against her mother. She was a completely normal individual until the age of 15½, at which time she noted that she had not started to menstruate, although all her girl friends had. She went to a physician who gave her capsules. This was followed shortly by a menstrual period and by a spontaneous period a month later. Shortly after this, in her 16th year, she met her first real boy friend. He was approximately the same age as she and they were quite in love with each other, promising marriage. Sexual activities with this boy were limited to kissing and holding each other's hands. There were many fantasies connected with this boy, all of a very romantic nature. None of them went beyond the act of kissing, but she states that she got a tremendous thrill even out of these fantasies. This boy could not hold a job and he was very distasteful to the patient's parents, who intimidated her and threatened dire consequences if she contined to go with him. During the first month of this relationship, the boy was acceptable to the parents, but at this time there arose a dispute between the boy and pt.'s mother. Angry words flew and from then on her parents would have absolutely nothing to do with the boy and disliked him intensely. However, this relationship lasted one year, the last few months of which the pt.'s mother often visited the parents of the boy and threatened them that she would kill herself if they did not tell their son to abstain from seeing her daughter. At the wish of her parents, pt. finally gave up this boy friend. Immediately thereafter she confined her activities to the house almost exclusively; she ate excessively and continually for several months, gaining about 15 pounds.

During this time her parents introduced her to an older man, about ten years older than herself, whom they wished her to marry. This man was very distasteful to her physically as well as as regards his personality. He was urged upon her with the statements that he had character and excellent standing and a good family. After going with him for about a month, he attempted sexual advances which disgusted and nauseated her. (N.B.: When she first met him and he was physically distasteful, she used to allude to him as her father or her grandfather.) She then went to see a doctor because of her overweight. He took a BMR and told her that her thyroid gland was not functioning and gave her thyroid medication and a diet. This resulted in loss of weight and about five months ago, she discontinued the thyroid tablets and the diet as she had been satisfied with the loss. However, she continued to lose weight, going from about 114 to 84 pounds in two months. During this time, her wedding with the older man has been postponed until she is physically fit. She states that the attentions of her fiance leave her completely cold emotionally and sexually, that his slightest physical advance, such as placing his arm around her, makes her shudder. Yet she states that she is in love with him, realiaing that he has stuck by her during her illness as no one else has or would.

Figure 4.1 Dr. Waller's clinical notes, October 24, 1938.

The home life of the pt. has always been marked by fights and squabbles. Her mother has continually nagged at her and her father frequently flies into a temper, particularly "if things do not go smoothly at home." The relationship between mother and father seems to be good, marked with very little strife. There are two younger brothers, 15 and 11 years of age. When the pt. was at High School, she did very well in her studies; yet she was constantly nagged by her mother to do her home-work and be proficient in school. Shortly after graduation, she began to feel a distinct inferiority both for herself and her entire family, as regards the neighbors and friends. This inferiority embraced personality factors as well as intelligence. She felt that she was dumb and particularly that her two brothers were dumb. The thoughts are still present. The 15 year old brother should be a man by now, yet he is very happy-go-lucky and is not good at school. The younger brother is very shy and refuses to go out to meet people. These thoughts bother her and take up a great deal of her time. The inferiority also embraces the mother and father.

Statement regarding the mother: The mother was very anxious to know what the daughter had said. She stated that her daughter had always fought with her; as long as she could remember, they had never agreed about anything. She could not understand this because she had been so good to her. She stated that her first boy friend was a tramp, came from a very poor family, and had no financial backing or future. He could not hold a job and had an awful temper. She also stated she could not understand why her daughter went with him and was so attached to him, because the two were always fighting. She is very desirous that her daughter marry the man with whom she is now going as he is very acceptable, but she wants to know whether or not her daughter loves him, as she feels that that is the primary consideration, and she would not insist on matrimony against her daughter's wishes. At present, mother is terribly worried that the same cycle of refusal to eat and loss of weight has started again, since the patient is out of the hospital. At this interview, the mother was advised that the only path for her to follow at the present time was to completely refrain from influencing the daughter's daily life: to allow her to eat or not as she pleases, sleep or not as she plases, go out of the house or not as she pleases. If the mother's advice is asked, she should make no definite answer, but say, It is up to you.

Dr. John Waller

October 31, 1938
Patient is pre-occupied with thoughts of her mother and the conflict which is constantly present between them and which has become worse in the past few months. The mother spends the greater part of the day lying on her bed, crying, and stating that she has given up all hope for the daughter's cure and that she herself would be better off dead. (Patient feels that if she did get better, it would not make any difference to the mother, because she would find something else wrong with the patient. All her life mother has found something wrong with her and she will probably continue to do so for the rest of her life.) When asked as to her reaction to her mother's death thoughts the patient shows strong emotional reaction and weeps whenever the subject is brought up. Indirect questioning fails to reveal any fantasies or wishes for the mother's death, but the patient states that should her mother die, she herself would commit suicide. The mother's expression of her death wish and the daugher's thoughts of suicide have been present for many years with the present accentuation only during the past few months. Apparently the mother has usedthis as one form of threat whenever a conflict or discussion arose between her and her daughter.

During the present illness patient did not eat because she wanted to lose weight. Then after losing a great deal of weight, she found that her appetite was completely gone. Since then, her appetite has returned, but the patient did not eat at first because she was afraid of constipation and a feeling of fullness. Constipation is a fear of the patient which has been present since childhood. She states she is afriad of constipation

Figure 4.2 Dr. Waller's clinical notes, October 24 and 31, 1938.

From the very beginning of their engagement, Waller's notes reflect the incompatibility of the mother–daughter relationship. "Mother wants to be good to me, but she would also like me dead." Ms. B considered "everything normal" until she was about 15 ½ (the same age as mother when she came to United States). Ms. B believed herself "different" from other girls who were menstruating (she was not) and began to feel others, including her family, did not like her. At 16, she began to have her "first real boyfriend," who was profoundly disapproved of by mother.

O. P. D. 23

NAME [redacted] page 2 NO. 52687 A

because she is afraid of getting piles and that her mother developed piles when she was pregnant with the patient. The other reason she has not eaten since the return of her appetite some months ago has been the actual presence of her mother, who, even if she says nothing, patient knows is constantly thinking about her and wishing that she would eat. If the patient goes to a restaurant where she is away from the family, she can and does eat a normal meal. The pregnancies of the mother with the second and third children are not recalled by the patient, but she states that the only time in her life when she was happy was shortly after the birth of the third child, when he was sick for a period of months with paroxysms of fainting and turning blue. The reason for her happiness was that her mother's attentions for that brief period were diverted from her to the sick child. Aside from this brief period, patient has suffered from excessive maternal care and anxiety which have played every move she has made.

At the age of 15-16 she became very friendly with a girl of her own age, spending the better part of her spare time with her, eating at her house and sleeping at her house. Mother and father objected very strenuously to this. Again the death wishes of the mother were expressed. After the parental influence had succeeded in breaking up this relationship, it was again successful in breaking up the relationship with her first boy friend. Prior to this first episode the patient cannot remember specific details of maternal conflict. She states that she always ate well and hence there was no maternal apprehension on that score. She also remembers nothing of the mother's pregnancies and has heard of no gastric disturbances or any other disease connected with the mother, except the piles which occurred during mother's first pregnancy.

When the patient was asked if she had any insight into her life story as so far presented and the development of her present illness, she stated that she guessed her under-eating was due to her conflict with her mother, since her appetite had returned several months ago. It was explained to her that she would react in a gastro-intestinal manner, probably because her mother had developed the piles which she feared so greatly herself, and, secondly, because of her mother's attention to her diet, and that her over-eating after the necessary rejection of the first boy friend was a reaction against the mother and that the mother did not want her to gain and in some way satisfied the romantic idea which had been associated with this boy friend. It was also explained that her refusal to eat and loss of appetite had accomplished two things, one being the production of a physical disease which would make her unacceptable to the fiance placed on her by her parents, and, secondly, a direct attack against the mother because mother wanted her to gain weight.

Patient seemed quite cheerful at the close of the session, expressed profuse thanks and seemed to be quite happy about the development of the picture.

Dr. John Waller

November 7, 1938
Patient entered, appearing quite happy and showing marked gain in weight. Relations with mother have been very amicable during the past week. Mother has not been nagging her verbally and there have been no more death wishes expressed on mother's part. However, patient feels that mother is continually thinking about her and nagging at her mentally, if not overtly. Patient has been eating well, particularly between meals and when away from home. Her appetite at home is still very poor. When questioned further as to her reaction to her mother's death wishes, there is no longer any emotional display. Her

Figure 4.3 Dr. Waller's clinical notes, October 31 and November 7, 1938.

Relationships worsened, mother "threatening to kill herself" if the relationship continued. Significantly, Ms. B dates the onset of her eating problems to this time, first "eating voraciously" over several months, with a weight gain of about 15 pounds. In the meantime, "mother's choice" for her was a man 10 years her senior that Ms. B found unappealing. Her weight then plummeted from 118 to 82, prompting mother to take her to medical clinic, where she was prescribed thyroid extract. Ms. B was more receptive to this older man when she was sick, finding him

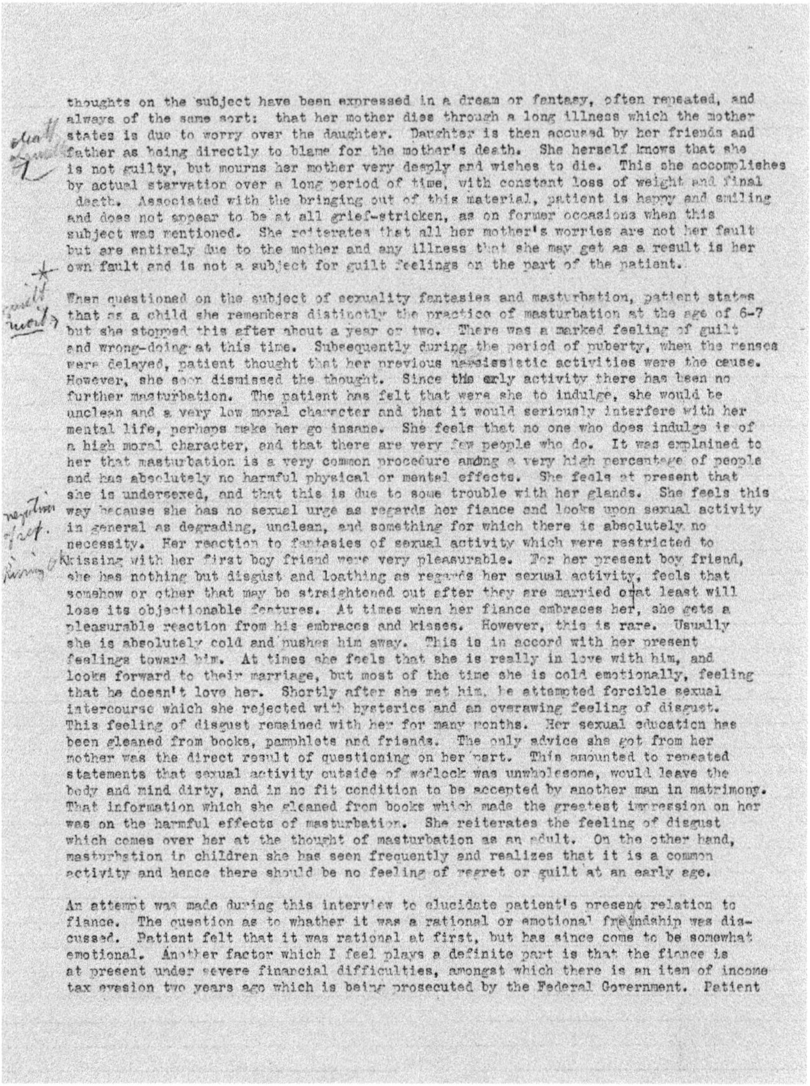

thoughts on the subject have been expressed in a dream or fantasy, often repeated, and always of the same sort: that her mother dies through a long illness which the mother states is due to worry over the daughter. Daughter is then accused by her friends and father as being directly to blame for the mother's death. She herself knows that she is not guilty, but mourns her mother very deeply and wishes to die. This she accomplishes by actual starvation over a long period of time, with constant loss of weight and final death. Associated with the bringing out of this material, patient is happy and smiling and does not appear to be at all grief-stricken, as on former occasions when this subject was mentioned. She reiterates that all her mother's worries are not her fault but are entirely due to the mother and any illness that she may get as a result is her own fault and is not a subject for guilt feelings on the part of the patient.

When questioned on the subject of sexuality fantasies and masturbation, patient states that as a child she remembers distinctly the practice of masturbation at the age of 6-7 but she stopped this after about a year or two. There was a marked feeling of guilt and wrong-doing at this time. Subsequently during the period of puberty, when the menses were delayed, patient thought that her previous narcissistic activities were the cause. However, she soon dismissed the thought. Since this early activity there has been no further masturbation. The patient has felt that were she to indulge, she would be unclean and a very low moral character and that it would seriously interfere with her mental life, perhaps make her go insane. She feels that no one who does indulge is of a high moral character, and that there are very few people who do. It was explained to her that masturbation is a very common procedure among a very high percentage of people and has absolutely no harmful physical or mental effects. She feels at present that she is undersexed, and that this is due to some trouble with her glands. She feels this way because she has no sexual urge as regards her fiance and looks upon sexual activity in general as degrading, unclean, and something for which there is absolutely no necessity. Her reaction to fantasies of sexual activity which were restricted to kissing with her first boy friend were very pleasurable. For her present boy friend, she has nothing but disgust and loathing as regards her sexual activity, feels that somehow or other that may be straightened out after they are married or at least will lose its objectionable features. At times when her fiance embraces her, she gets a pleasurable reaction from his embraces and kisses. However, this is rare. Usually she is absolutely cold and pushes him away. This is in accord with her present feelings toward him. At times she feels that she is really in love with him, and looks forward to their marriage, but most of the time she is cold emotionally, feeling that he doesn't love her. Shortly after she met him, he attempted forcible sexual intercourse which she rejected with hysterics and an overawing feeling of disgust. This feeling of disgust remained with her for many months. Her sexual education has been gleaned from books, pamphlets and friends. The only advice she got from her mother was the direct result of questioning on her part. This amounted to repeated statements that sexual activity outside of wedlock was unwholesome, would leave the body and mind dirty, and in no fit condition to be accepted by another man in matrimony. That information which she gleaned from books which made the greatest impression on her was on the harmful effects of masturbation. She reiterates the feeling of disgust which comes over her at the thought of masturbation as an adult. On the other hand, masturbation in children she has seen frequently and realizes that it is a common activity and hence there should be no feeling of regret or guilt at an early age.

An attempt was made during this interview to elucidate patient's present relation to fiance. The question as to whether it was a rational or emotional friendship was discussed. Patient felt that it was rational at first, but has since come to be somewhat emotional. Another factor which I feel plays a definite part is that the fiance is at present under severe financial difficulties, amongst which there is an item of income tax evasion two years ago which is being prosecuted by the Federal Government. Patient

Figure 4.4 Dr. Waller's clinical notes, November 7, 1938.

"more attentive" at those times. Such dramatic weight loss warranted hospitalization, and on Ms. B's discharge after a modest weight gain, mother was advised to "let her alone, to do as she wishes."

This did not alter things, and they became locked in a mutually destructive dyadic relationship, each threatening homicide or suicide. Eating problems persisted with "fears of fullness, constipation and piles" ("like mother had during pregnancy" with daughter). Therapist clarified that not eating was a way of gaining revenge on mother for aborting the

O. P. D. 23

NAME [redacted] page 3 NO 52687A

states that as long as financial difficulties are present, matrimony is out of the question. Her parents still feel very kindly towards the fiance, hope and think that his financial difficulties will be straightened out in short order and look forward to the wedding. They, of course, would not accept him at the present moment. Patient showed a very marked ignorance as regards the sexual aspect of marital life. She was advised to talk things over with one of her recently married cousins.

Dr. John Waller

November 21, 1938

Patient is in good spirits but complains bitterly of a recent change in habits. Of late she has been turning night into day, and vice versa. She goes to bed anywhere from 3-7 a.m., sleeps almost all day. Stays up at night and eats everything in sight. She does not start eating until after her parents have gone to bed. She then proceeds, not out of hunger, but just because she wants something to do, to eat. The list includes many things for which she formerly had no desire. The process of eating continues until she feels upper abdominal pain and still she continues to eat, paying no attention to the pain, and she states that her stomach feels tremendous and heavy, as though it were sticking way out. This does not deter her from further eating, until such time as she chooses to go to bed. During the day time and when her parents, particularly her mother, are ~~not~~ in evidence, she eats very little. If, however, she goes to a restaurant during the day, she gorges herself much the same as she does at home at night. The feeling of abdominal pain and distention and largeness are related to the sensation of pregnancy. She has had fantasies of pregnancy, always associated with the same abdominal pain and feeling of distention. During these fantasies she is terribly worried about pregnancy, chiefly because of the fear of discomfort and labor. In these dreams of pregnancy, she has wondered why her child has no father. There has been a complete absence of fantasy as regards the paternal side. On one occasion she gave birth to a baby boy. There was no labor fantasy connected with this, merely the fact that she was pregnant and that afterwards she had the baby boy. With all the eating the patient is doing at the present time, there is severe constipation, for which she takes repeated cathartics.

The patient's knowledge of pregnancy and the complications of pregnancy were gathered from books on the subject and conversations with friends, both those who have been and have not been pregnant. She knows that her mother suffered severely during labor when the patient's two younger brothers were born. However she does not know of any GI disturbance during any of her mother's three pregnancies.

Patient's relationship with her fiance has improved. She welcomes his kisses and embraces, but still feels that when they are married, sexual intercourse will be abhorrent. This she believes is connected with her fear of pregnancy and labor, although she very much wants to have a child. She is completely without hope for the future since she feels that financial circumstances are such and will continue to be such that she cannot get married. All social intercourse with friends and relatives has been discontinued. Patient feels absolutely no desire to see any of them. She states that she felt a maternal aunt, the aunt's husband and daughter, had a great deal to do with her PI, that their curses and jealousy brought on her lack of appetite and malnutrition. She states she knows that is ridiculous, but she cannot help feeling it at times.

Figure 4.5 Dr. Waller's clinical notes, November 7 and 21, 1938.

relationship with first boyfriend. In a session after this clarification/interpretation, "warfare" between mother and daughter "cooled down," death threats ceased (temporarily), but Ms. B soon dreamed of mother dying, feeling blamed but not guilty.

Association with her "older" fiancé is marked with increased eating, "until very full, like pregnancy." Discussion about marriage by the therapist raised issues of masturbation and repulsion of intercourse although she "wants to have a baby." She believed that children were born only in

O. P. D. 23

NAME [redacted] page 8 NO.

February 21, 1939
Patient came alone, for the first time. Had a scrap with her mother about eating and told her she was going to a show. Patient came to the hospital anyway, or she just wanted to punish her mother.

conflict c̄ mother

All her life the patient has felt it necessary to make life miserable for her mother, but each act has also been calculated to hurt herself. She has a very guilty feeling about hurting her mother and during the interview cries when talking about it.

Every friend the patient has, or relative, she either likes or dislikes only on the basis of their reaction to her. Even with her first boy friend, she did not love him until he declared his love. It has always been this way and the patient thinks this is because she is selfish.

A recent dream: she married her discarded fiance and went to bed with him with great fright. When she awoke it was her maternal uncle she had married. This was repulsive and she felt it a terrible thing to have to go through life married to an older man.

February 28, 1939
During the past week there has been a return of spontaneous crying and nervousness, despite the fact that the open conflict with the mother is somewhat less frequent and violent. The patient's appetite is still almost nil, and she thinks she is losing weight. Even the occasional appetite she has does not increase her food intake because she is afraid of constipation.

Dates with boys have been discouraged by the patient, since she is afraid to go out with them, afraid for two reasons: (1) she may be attacked and will not know how to take care of sexual approaches, (2) that her pride would be hurt too much if a boy did not ask her for another date.

I am apparently unable to get to the basis of this neurosis and on Dr. Kaufman's advice, will attempt to turn the patient over to Dr. Jessner Monday morning.
Dr. John Waller.

March 6, 1939
Patient is not feeling well and has repeated episodes of nervousness. Open conflicts with her mother are not so frequent. She will not go out with boys, as she is afraid of being attacked. When asked about herthoughts about myself, she states that I would not attack her because I am a doctor, that during the day she thinks about everybody, that I am included, as is Dr. Kaufman. If I had a date with her outside of professional relations, I would attack her, as well as would any other man she went out with.

Figure 4.6 Dr. Waller's clinical notes, February 21 and 28 and March 6, 1939.

wedlock, yet she "abhors the idea of intercourse," even in marriage. In one dream, she sees fiancé, who "turns out to be maternal uncle." Little seems made of this dream by her therapist.

In the sessions between November 30, 1938 and February 14, 1939 (facsimile omitted), the vacillating pattern of mother–daughter squabbling, anger and physical violence persist.

Several sessions brought out additional sexual history, relationship to father and more conflict over relationship to fiancé of "older man."

She believed she obtained sexual knowledge from books and friends. At age 6, she thought that kissing led to pregnancy but had no other thoughts about it. Childhood sex play ("playing house") existed with friends and later with brothers. Not until 12 did she learn about menstruation and intercourse from her girlfriend and was disgusted to understand that parents "did it." During the early years, she "slept more in their bed than her own." At 16, her boyfriend disgusted her with a description of fellatio. She could admit that she was "sexually thrilled when her early boyfriend kissed her." Few dreams are reported during her sessions, although in one she is chased by men with knives. In another, she dreams of Errol Flynn "making love" to her and being thrilled by his embrace. (At the time, Flynn was not only a popular swashbuckling movie actor in the 1930s but also a known philanderer, giving rise to the expression "in like Flynn.") Bedwetting "until junior high school" was acknowledged.

In the new year (1939), Ms. B reported feeling in good spirits, also denying that she was "ever very sick, except for the weight loss." Compulsions, she says, have subsided. Her weight remains steady around 104–106 for several sessions. In the January 17 session, Dr. Waller arranged a consultation with Dr. Kaufman, who consults with therapist and patient the next week. She revealed to Dr. Kaufman that when her first brother was born, she was "jealous of his closeness to mother's breast." She thought that with his birth, she became father's favorite while the new baby was mother's. She thought "how nice it would be if she could go away with father and take mother's place." Acknowledging that the "older man" that mother "forced on her" reminded her of father elicited the comment that "incest is unacceptable." (This is a rare glimpse of fantasies about father and not entirely clear how much is reflected in the patient's own words, Dr. Kaufman's remarks, or the therapist's translation of all that is said between them.) Someone is quoted as saying "compulsive eating was compensation for sexual gratification." Her solution, probably attributed to Kaufman, was "to revert to childhood and thereby have control over her parents." (The issue of whose reality is expressed in some of the data reported in this case is evident in the topic of "oral impregnation" [discussed later].) Such fantasy is not attributed to the patient in Dr. Waller's notes but seems to have been assumed by the therapist himself. Her therapist states in the December 30 session that "going to bed after eating is related to ideas of eating and pregnancy and intercourse."

In the session after Dr. Kaufman's participation, Ms. B reported feeling better and was noted by therapist to be "in pretty good spirits," that "things at home were much better the past week." She thought her "reaction to mother was in large part jealousy for the father." (Did Kaufman's "interpretive" comments awaken some degree of insight in Ms. B?)

Curiously, this fleeting apparent "insight" was followed by missing her next session. In her place, mother appeared, confirming that the patient's "condition is much better towards the family," that she is "much more considerate of my ill health," but compulsions continue nonetheless and Ms. B persists in her belief that "she will never get well as long as I am alive."

During her next session, on February 8, the patient seems to revert to old habits of sleeping and eating, while weight remains around 106. She guiltily states that mother's illness is probably her fault. The session seems rather fallow and Dr. Waller is moved to resurrect the post-Kaufman "improvement" by telling her that "when she had arrived at a fundamental understanding of the material which had been brought forth previously," she would "no longer react to mother as she has in the past."

A session was held on February 14, but no mention is made of Valentine's Day. Notes indicate, however, that this is "the first time she has come in without makeup." (Therapist seems not to comment on transference implications.) She appears depressed and says that she and her mother "are children" and that "all my family are immature, except my father." The therapist concludes the session by suggesting that perhaps she should go away to visit relatives in New York for a couple of weeks (possibly his way of reacting to subtle evidence of discomfiting positive transference). Her response is that they would try to introduce her to men who would take advantage of her and "sell her into white slavery."

When Ms. B misses an occasional appointment, mother comes to the therapist, complains about her daughter's waxing and waning rituals, seemingly related to visits by her fiancé. Mother describes how the outbursts of temper cause her to wish she herself were dead and that the two of them would die and be buried together. Mother describes how daughter is affectionate toward her when she is sick, tells mother "my heart isn't made of stone." But then mother states that her daughter must be "insane" to have such opposing attitudes. Dr. Waller "reassures" mother her daughter is "not crazy" but then states that her daughter will be "100% cured" (perhaps a need to reassure himself in situations that seem hopeless).

The emphasis through most sessions is reflected in Waller's notes from the very first visit that "there is an open conflict between the family and the patient…particularly true of the mother-daughter relationship."

In spite of the poor outcome reported by Waller, the case generated considerable interest in subsequent reports of anorexia and was the likely source of several citations: Deutsch's demonstration of his associative anamnesis (Deutsch, 1939), the patient example in the paper by Waller with Kaufman and Deutsch (1940) and evidence of a presentation by Deutsch to a psychoanalytic audience. Much later, I described the patient in my 1989 paper in *Psychosomatic Medicine* (Lipsitt, 1989).

Around this time, Dr. Deutsch demonstrated his interview technique with Ms. B.

Dr. Deutsch's Encounter with Ms. B (Exact Date Unknown)

Dr. Felix Deutsch's comments and interview with Ms. B and his Associative Anamnesis are reproduced here [unedited] in their entirety (Deutsch, 1939).

> The patient is a nineteen-year-old salesgirl, born in this country of European parents. Her chief complaint on admission was loss of weight. About one year ago the patient weighed one hundred eighteen pounds and at that time began to eat compulsively all sorts of pastries and sweets and soon put on twenty pounds, after which she consulted a physician because she was overweight.
>
> Because her basal metabolic rate was –28 she was put on thyroid medication. After the loss of twenty pounds her basal metabolic rate was still –28 and when she reached one hundred and fourteen pounds the thyroid was stopped. However, the patient could not eat. She complained of loss of appetite and a great aversion to food. She then stopped eating altogether and noticed that she drank a great deal of water, perhaps sixteen glasses a day. This was not because she was thirsty, but because she had to do something to keep things out of her mind. During the period when she had put on twenty pounds and was eating compulsively, she stated that she did not eat because she was hungry but also 'to keep things away from my mind'. At the time of admission her weight was eighty-seven and one-half pounds. She gave a history of constipation dating back to her childhood and gave this as one of the reasons for her lack of appetite. She complained of weakness and irritability, with an intensification of quarreling with her parents.
>
> At the age of fifteen, as her menses had not appeared, oral endocrine therapy was resorted to and this was followed by two scanty periods one month apart. Since that time she had had no menstrual periods. A year later this medication was repeated and another scanty flow resulted. Since that time she has had no menstrual periods. Related to her large fluid intake there was frequent and copious urination.
>
> Physical examination revealed an emaciated girl who appeared alert and intelligent and gave no evidence of distress. She was heavily made up, with rouged cheeks and lips and penciled eyebrows.
>
> Her breasts were well developed in spite of the recent extreme loss of weight. There was a marked hirsutism over the whole body, particularly over the arms and legs, which the patient attributed to the use of a depilatory.
>
> A thorough physical examination, including x-rays of the skull and chest, and laboratory tests, was completely normal. There was no evidence of hyperthyroidism. The ward diagnoses were: Simmonds' disease, diabetes insipidus, or anorexia nervosa.

The Associative Anamnesis

DR: I wanted to know about your illness.

PT: You don't know anything about me? Oh gosh. Well, I am here because I am a hypo something or other. My thyroid. I have lost a lot of weight in the past few months. I am all run down, and so forth, and so forth. Hasn't my record been sent down here?

DR: Are you so well trained to talk in medical terms?

PT: I am a doctor (laughs). I hear all the doctors talking about it, so I learned it from them, all the doctors upstairs. They said I was a hypo something or other. I don't know, and I had lost a lot of weight, and I am here to gain it and have myself all cured, I guess. I was sent here; I didn't come myself. I was in the endocrine department and I saw a doctor there and he said I had to go to the hospital because I kept on losing weight. When I first came I weighed one hundred and two, the next time ninety-nine, and the next ninety-two, and the fourth time, eighty-five, so he said to go to the hospital because I couldn't lose any more weight.

DR: What do you think about losing weight?

PT: I don't know. I haven't been eating enough. I was on a diet from before and I guess my stomach shrunk. I didn't feel like eating after that and when I tried to, it didn't do any good. My nerves were so bad and whenever I sat down to eat, I got so nervous that I couldn't eat. I almost wanted to kill myself, I didn't know what to do, because I was so skinny and I gave everyone a pain in the neck. I have been here a few days and I feel much better. I kept on losing weight and over here I think I gained some weight already.

DR: Eating was so difficult?

PT: I don't know. Everything was so hard. I didn't enjoy anything. My heart would start beating fast and I felt as if my heart would go away from me. I kept on losing that weight and the doctor said I could not afford to lose any more, so he sent me into the hospital.

DR: Could not eat?

PT: I could a little, but not much. Since I have been like this, I got hair all over my body, fine hair, and the hair on my head keeps falling out and falling out.

DR: And you could not eat?

PT: I could a little, but not much. I was on a diet before because I was fatter and I wanted to get thin. A few months ago, in March, I weighed one hundred and thirty-eight. I was ashamed of myself because I was too fat. I took some of those thyroid pills and they made me thin too. But when I stopped taking the pills, I kept on going down and down. I used to get chills in my head, all around, used to feel the wind in my head going round and round. Inside, the wind like chills going in my head; then all over my body. I used to shiver, then I would feel hot in my head and feel hot all over. And the hair I got. I never had that before. That just started recently, on my arms and all over.

DR: You did not want to be fat?

PT: I was too stout. I used to eat too much. Every minute I used to eat, because I didn't care what happened to me. Ate and ate and ate and ate, and then gained so much that I was ashamed. All my clothes were too tight and I didn't want to buy new clothes.

DR: Ashamed to eat?

PT: No, ashamed to be stout. I don't know what else.

DR: What?

PT: I am very constipated. I don't move my bowels. It is very hard for me to move my bowels. But I feel a little better since I have been here. I came Saturday and I think I gained some weight too. I have to force the food in my stomach and they give me a very fattening diet here.

DR: Who told you to eat every minute?

PT: Myself. I told myself because I didn't care about anything. I used to sit in the house all day long, never wanted to go out, and when I woke up, I used to start eating until I went to bed. All kinds of candies and cakes and pies and every minute my mouth used to be working. You know, chewing food. Suddenly I became ashamed. So I went all the way down to eighty-five. Now I think I weigh ninety.

DR: You liked to eat.

PT: Then I did. But now when I have to eat, I get nervous.

DR: What do you mean?

PT: Inside, I sort of feel afraid, as soon as I have to start eating. After I eat, I feel a little better. I don't know why I am afraid, but I get nervous. Everything starts to jump inside and I. feel like crying when I have to go and eat. [Cries]

DR: Why should you cry?

PT: Because I have not eaten so much for so long. I just ate a little. Here they give me so much and I am not used to it. So I feel like crying.

DR: You cry often?

PT: When I was nervous and sick I did. Lately, before, when I was healthy, I never used to cry. When I was healthy I always wanted to eat very much. Now I would still like to eat, but I am sort of afraid. I don't know why: I don't know what it is. I am afraid I will be constipated and my bowels will not work. I don't know. I don't know what it is. Maybe because a year ago I used to overeat so much that I gained so much and went up to a hundred and thirty-eight. My normal weight is a hundred and eighteen. So maybe now I am afraid of overeating. Still I want to get fat. I want to weigh about one hundred fifteen or one hundred eighteen, but still I am afraid and then I am afraid I will be constipated.

DR: When you eat, you are afraid?

PT: When I have to go, when they say, 'Here is your food', I start to get nervous. That fright comes over me a little bit. At home I was crying every minute and yelled at everyone. I didn't mean it, but I yelled. I used to call my mother names. Honestly. Because she used to tell me to eat. She used to yell at me because I didn't eat and then I would yell back at her and then I would go into my room and start crying because I yelled at her.

DR: You cried because you yelled at her?

PT: I used to yell at my father and brother and boyfriend and I didn't want to go anywhere, dances or parties. I wanted to stay home all the time. I was so nervous. But I have so many enemies because I used to fight with them. I didn't mean it, but I was so nervous that I couldn't control myself. I used to say things to them that would hurt them. On account of that I don't think anyone likes me now. I got so nervous and upset that I would say anything. My mother would say something to me, if she was mad, like 'I want you to get out of this house', or, 'I hate you', or, 'I don't want to see you before my eyes any more', and I used to say the same things back to her. I said the same things, although I didn't mean them. She said these things because I didn't eat and she got disgusted. She wanted me to gain weight and I was losing. So that is the story. As soon as she would tell me to eat, I used to get so nervous and then I could not eat, and she yelled at me and I yelled back at her. We have so many arguments all the time. In any little thing we had arguments. My mother is too good to me. She brought me up in the wrong way. She gave me everything I wanted and even things I didn't want. Not that she could afford them, but little things. She was too good to me. So I said anything to her and she would not answer me back. If I ever started to yell, she didn't hit me for yelling at her, so I think she brought me up in the wrong way. Too good to me.

DR: Too good to you.

PT: She always wanted me to eat, but when I was fat, then she didn't want me to eat so much because I ate too much then. She said that I ate too much and was too fat. She only said that once in a while; she didn't want me to gain more weight. (Cries.)

DR: You are unhappy.

PT: No, I have a lump in my throat and I have to relieve it.

DR: By crying?

PT: That is the only way. Otherwise it chokes me. When I try to control myself, it doesn't do any good. I cannot control myself. I try and try, but I just can't.

DR: You can cry?

PT: Yes, but nothing bothers me now. I don't know what it is. Nerves, my nerves must be very weak.

DR: Something did bother you?

PT: No. Well, I did feel a little bad before. A certain nurse here, she says, 'You have to do this and you have to do that'. Every time she talks to me she never smiles, just says, 'You have to drink that by ten o'clock'. What difference does it make if I drink it five minutes after ten? But everything right now bothers me; otherwise I wouldn't mind it.

DR: All that started in March?

PT: It began when I was losing weight. Started to get worse and worse. First I was normal and then I used to overeat until I became fat and then I went all the way down to now. But I feel a little better now than when I first came.

DR: You were always yelling at everyone.

PT: Yes, I was, Because I was nervous, so I yelled at anyone. My friends, my boyfriend, and girl friends and parents.

DR: Your boyfriend?

PT: I said things he didn't like and I used to yell.

DR: Who yelled in the house?

PT: I don't know. I did most of the yelling. And then everyone yelled at me because I yelled at them. Then I was hurt and felt badly and there was a whole mix-up. Yelled at my mother and father.

DR: Father yelled too?

PT: Oh yes, sure. He always used to yell. Even before I was sick. If I did something he didn't want me to. Now everyone yells too.

DR: He yelled at mother also?

PT: Once in a while. But I think everyone yells. He didn't yell at her often, did not want to think, so I ate.

DR: All that came on suddenly.

PT: Not suddenly, because I was on a diet and I was taking thyroid. It started about March. Before that, I ate too much and then not enough.

DR: How long did you eat too much?

PT: September, October, November, December, January, February, so much. October, it wasn't so bad, but went real good in January and February. I wanted to eat all the time. To have something in my mouth so that I would be occupied, doing something. I did not want to think, so I used to eat. My mother made me stop going with a boy, so I used to eat to keep myself from thinking. She didn't like him; he was no good. Every time he had a job, he used to quit and he would not work. So she didn't want me to go with a boy like that. I liked him very much. I know that I shouldn't, but I couldn't help it. I knew that he would not make a good husband, because he always changed his mind and his job. Every month he had another job. That is not good. But I liked him and I couldn't stop seeing him. Now I am happy that I stopped going with him, because if I married him, I would not have a good husband, and now I have my own boyfriend, another one. A nice boy. I knew him since September and I didn't like him at first, although my parents liked him. I didn't like him until two months ago. I went with him because my parents said he was a wonderful person. I went with him on account of them. But now I really love him. At the beginning it was terrible. I used to fight with my parents. I used to say, 'I am not in love with him'. And they said that I should keep on seeing him. I didn't care for him. He is ten years older, very settled, more serious, and, I don't know, I just didn't feel akin to him. But I kept on going with him because he was crazy about me. I was a pretty girl then. Now I really love him. But it certainly took me a long time and a lot of suffering, because first I got fat and then I didn't eat enough and now I am trying to get back to normal.

DR: The other boy was your age.

PT: Two years older. Yes, nearer my age. He liked what I liked and he was crazy about me. He was more emotional. This one is also emotional and especially in his approach to me, but the other was more impulsive, more impulsive in his actions. If he wanted to do something he would do it. Very impetuous, very hasty. He would give me a push and then take me in his arms and kiss me. He was tall and husky. But he would not make a good husband; I realize that now. He is all right to see once in a while for amusement, but not to marry. This boy is just the opposite, quiet, settled, reserved, and sure about his job. The other one didn't care. If he lost his job, he lost it. But this one is so kind to me, very patient with me, because I yelled at him so much and told him to go and that I didn't want to see him anymore. He knows I am nervous, so he comes back, and he has been very good to me. I have been going with him for a whole year. He kisses me too and takes me around, but he is different. I don't feel those emotions for him. He was here to see me this afternoon. If it was any other boy, well, I got so homely. I used to be pretty, but I kept on losing weight, but he kept on seeing me. He hopes now and my mother hopes now.

DR: And you hope?

PT: I hope too. I want to be pretty as I used to be and happy. At first I didn't care because I was so skinny; I didn't even care for my boyfriend. But now I want to get normal. I don't want to be so nervous and irritable. Everything changed. My hair was oily and thick and now it is so dry and falling out; hair on my hands, I never had it like that. And on my body too.

DR: You could never eat when you were upset?

PT: No, when I was upset I could always eat. Everyone always used to say, 'When I get nervous, I cannot eat', and I could always eat all the time. Then it changed.

DR: Mother reacted in this way too?

PT: Sure, lots of times. When she was arguing with my father or me, she did not eat. She felt disgusted and did not want to eat. Whenever she was disgusted, she could not eat.

DR: Nor drink?

PT: I don't know about drinking. But she would drink straight water. I can drink water even when I am nervous. Sometimes it sort of comes up. I feel it but I force it down. When I am nervous, I have to force something to eat or drink.

DR: Thank you. I will see you again. [Not clear that he did!—au.]

Dr. Deutsch's Summary

> The associative anamnesis of this patient contains the highlights of the psychosomatic symptom complex called anorexia nervosa: the specific eating problem, the functional disorders of the intestines, the endocrine dysfunctions, the characteristic sexual struggles, the family situation in different periods of life, and the interaction of the parental and patient's neuroses.

Author's comment: This interview by Dr. Deutsch in 1939 may not seem so different from a good psychiatric interview performed today (see interview by Dr. Eisendrath). Attention to "psychosomatic" elements in a patient's "wholeness" was just beginning to be appreciated at the time. The departure from a totally organic approach to disease was addressed by Deutsch as a "psychosomatic unit," with a focus on "the active or latent coordination of and interaction between a given organ and a psychic conflict" (Deutsch, 1959). This approach did not become fully incorporated into psychiatric evaluation and practice until many years later, especially with increasing adherents to the biopsychosocial model.

Dr. John Romano's Interview

Dr. Romano interviewed the patient in 1941 in what may have been several relatively brief contacts. Excerpts of Romano's clinical notes with Ms. B appear here. She was 21 at the time.

Dr. Romano, whether out of special interest or the patient's preoccupation, focused largely on somatic complaints. Dr. Romano's notes imply that he saw her more than two or three times, with extended interviews each time, mostly by herself, at times with the mother. On a first visit, on May 14, 1941, mother dated the patient's difficulties beginning 4 years prior, 1937.

According to mother, "she was a good girl when she was small, but she was wild." The only difficulty was in getting her to go to bed.

> She has supper and a few hours later she eats and eats and eats and drinks and drinks and then goes into the bathroom and when I get up in the middle of the night, she's asleep there in the bathroom.

Mother described her daughter as "stubborn, without any responsibilities." She said her daughter was "unbalanced; her veins is tied up (sic)." She admitted slapping the patient "for her own good." Sometimes the patient would come to mother's door and laugh and sing. When the patient screams, mother puts her hand over the patient's mouth and in the process scratches the patient's face with her fingernails. On one occasion, mother complained that her daughter allowed a girlfriend to comb her hair in her room while rejecting mother's efforts to do so. Much was alluded to of the patient's compulsive behaviors like shaking out her clothes repeatedly, wiping down furniture or removing exudate from her eyes. Mother's observation is that patient behaves this way at home but outside the house is quite different.

Mother was asked to leave the interview session when patient complained of her "interference." The patient then embarked on a long explanation of why she had to remove mucus from her eyes. "I have an awful lot of trouble with my head and my eyes; if I don't pull the mucus out, I get black circles under my eyes and a terrible headache." This condition keeps her from "going out" because of feelings of shame about needing to clear her eyes. "It makes me so miserable sometimes I feel as if I'm half dead. My head is so hazy I can't concentrate on anything and it seems as if I'm walking around half alive."

The patient said she was extremely nervous, starting about 3 years ago. She began to feel she was too fat from overeating and decided to diet, losing much weight from 138 to 82 pounds, at which time she was taken to a hospital for observation, continuing with much anxiety. "Everything excites me. When anybody would tell me to eat, my stomach would cramp up and I couldn't eat a thing." She cut down food intake more and more until she was eating "practically nothing."

In the BIH for 12 days, she gained 6 pounds. She said she was frightened when she got to 83 pounds but was strangely "glad inside." She did not want to get back to 138 pounds, and when she reached 90 pounds, she felt she still wanted to lose weight. On discharge, she had hopes of trying to hold her weight to the 118 she considered her normal, but "when her father, mother or boyfriend would order her to eat, she would have to stop eating and leave the table." For the next year, her weight remained in 90s.

When very thin, she would vomit. She would get heartburn and belch up "sour stuff" and have "belly pain." People would comment on how thin she looked. Expecting to attend an uncle's wedding, she wanted to gain some weight in order to not feel ashamed at the ceremony. She managed to gain about 10 pounds and did attend in an evening gown. She continued gaining weight afterwards.

She thought "all her sicknesses" came on when she was gaining weight, "not when I am losing it." Though "constipated as long as I can remember," on discharge from the hospital while gaining weight she had frequent episodes of diarrhea "with pains all over my body about 2 or 3 times a week." This would alternate with constipation for the next year, resulting in "piles and hemorrhoids" (like mother had).

Eating was erratic. Sometimes just milk and cake. Other times, it included cottage cheese, fruit, orange juice and occasional meat. At one time, her whole body had a yellow hue, believed to have come from drinking large quantities of carrot juice. Most of the time, she consumed large amounts of water. "I eat everything in one meal because we [mother] quarrel all day long and by the time I eat I'm starved." Eating may occur at any time of day (or night).

Sleep pattern is very erratic, going to bed in early morning hours, retiring at different times almost every day. "I forget that the clock is moving so I go to bed very late." Mother will find her asleep in the bathroom in the morning: "She argues with me about everything; she throws things at me and argues about going to bed late, but if not, then it's always something else."

Periods had not occurred for the past 3 ½ years (from 1937). She said it bothered her because "everybody has it except me." "Sometimes I think I won't be able to have children or anything like that." She claimed she would like to have children if she were normal, but she feels she is not normal; it is mostly her head and eyes and not having her period that bother her. Menstruation had begun at 15 or 16, ceasing after two periods, with two more a year later. Periods reduced in quantity over time with "only a few drops" and then ceased completely. She wondered if headaches were caused by lack of menstruating.

She continues to focus on physical symptoms. Much time is spent complaining of "red nose," which "makes me look like a freak," and keeps her from socializing with friends. She has feelings of heaviness around her sinuses, sore gums, nasal congestion, palpitations, sweating, edema of ankles, frequent urination, earache, and twitching of legs when sleeping. She has never had convulsions.

Tonsils and adenoids were removed when she was about 4. Her childhood illnesses included measles, mumps, chicken pox, German measles, whooping cough and scarlet fever. The only other surgery was "opening of my ear at about 5 or 6."

Dr. Romano's questions are largely not recorded, only the patient's responses. She goes on at length about abusive treatment from her mother and her brothers, not so much from father. He would argue with her but not hurt her physically. Mother

> pinches me or beats me with whatever she has in her hand or scratches me. I will be crying and after that I get dizzy and I don't know where I am. If she (mother) leaves the house when I am nervous I call her back and she does everything possible. She twists my nose and digs her nails into my face or hands. When she does that I hate her. Anything may start fights...usually going to bed late. She talks about it all day long.

She feels that brothers "have no respect for me at all, they treat me like a dog. They are so against me they are more like enemies of mine than like brothers. They never have a pleasant word for me." When speaking of her brothers, she would exhibit a kind of stuttering speech.

An oft-repeated theme appears prominently in Dr. Romano's notes. It concerns her many conflicts with parents about her boyfriend. She doesn't go with her boyfriend anymore. She broke off with him two years ago.

> At the beginning, I was going with him and I was a good normal weight and then I got too fat and went on a diet and went from 138 to 82 pounds and he didn't mind and was very nice to me. He wanted to get married but I didn't want to because I liked my former boyfriend that my parents were against. I gradually became accustomed to him (the one her parents liked) but I wasn't sure about marrying him. One time he tried to get fresh and I didn't let him. And then the next time nobody was home and he wanted to have intercourse. Because I was engaged and not married. I said I would maintain my standards. He tried to force me but he couldn't succeed because I struggled. He tried again later, we quarreled frequently about this and broke the engagement. He left and came back a week later. We had another quarrel and I told him to never set foot in my house again. It has been off for good since then.

The boy she liked had lived near her. They knew each other since she was 13. At 16 and 18, they began going together. He didn't ask her to have intercourse. "Sometimes he would get very passionate and I would push him off. He would kiss me and make love to me. I don't believe in intercourse unless you are married." Sometimes she dreams of intercourse with him, and if she were married, she thinks she would enjoy having intercourse with him. Sometimes when they are together, he would ejaculate. She didn't mind and almost enjoyed it as long as it wasn't intercourse. It made her "more tied to him." She made a distinction between semen and the mucus that comes out of her eyes. She knew "semen was how you had a child," and she was careful in cleaning it off. She added that she never feared impregnation just from kissing. Regarding marriage, she said

> I don't feel well lately though I would like to get married because it is the normal thing, but I feel so dizzy and suffer with my head and eyes, I feel that if I got married I would always be feeling bad and going to doctors and you can't get married on that basis. You have to be healthy.

Her parents, especially father, were against this boy. Her father was against him and would not let her go with him. "I don't know if it was puppy love or what, but we liked each other very much." Her father threatened her mother with divorce if she did not prevent her from seeing this boy. Father moved the family out of the neighborhood after making her break off with this boy (about 4 years ago, 1937, age 17). Her parents then urged her to go with a man (10 years her senior) that she did not like. One time in the car, he tried to stimulate her, but she wouldn't let him. He touched her but didn't "go into" her when she struggled and screamed. He asked her to stimulate him, took out his penis and tried to "put my hand on his penis but I didn't want to and I told him to stop and we quarreled on account of that." For the past 2 years, there has been no sexual activity, although she would occasionally stimulate herself.

She was about 11 when she first learned from a girlfriend about menstruation and about how babies were born. At first, she didn't believe it. "When this girl told me that babies are born by a man and a woman having intercourse I didn't want to believe that my parents had done that because I thought it was dirty." She recalled "playing house" or "hospital" as a 6-year-old when boys and girls would touch each other. She thinks a little boy tried to put his penis in her at the time, but she wouldn't let him. She said that brothers and father never got "fresh" with her.

Because of her "bad nature," she feels "as if I am walking around in a daze." Sometimes, when she quarrels with mother, she "doesn't care what she does and does everything to harm herself, eating junk food that is no good for her." One time she had a terrible fight with her mother in which "she almost crippled me." She cried all day and night and then started to eat, when mother came out to the kitchen, fought her and pinched her. She said her mother prayed to God that she (the daughter) would die. She sometimes feels she would like to die because she feels "so in between." She tried on one occasion to turn on the gas "to make mother free," but mother came and tuned it off.

Only 5 days later Dr. Romano again saw the patient, who had the usual repetition of physical complaints: headache, tiredness, mucus in eyes, athlete's foot, nervousness, carbuncle on chin, ulcer in cheek and red nose. She elaborated on her compulsivity and the need to repeatedly shake out her clothes "because they may have accumulated dust overnight." She checks the door frequently, wipes everything down (chairs, sink, etc.), and washes her hands until they are rough and raw.

This session included much more about the patient's eating habits.

> I made an awful habit to come home and sit down and eat. When I start I am so tired. I am too lazy to get up and go to bed. I'll sometimes read a little like physical culture, the dictionary, the encyclopedia articles about heart disease, but they say nothing about red noses or mucus in the eyes. I'll read my brother's detective stories or sometimes even my kid brother's comic books. While reading, I eat. Eat anything, cake, fruit, strawberries and cream, milk, all kinds of crazy conglomerations of food, one at a time.

This keeps her up a long time and then she gets sick because she has eaten so much junk. She then has to take something, either mineral oil or something. "Because I have a funny feeling from all that food, my stomach is bloated. My stomach usually comes out like that, awfully big from eating so much food." She feels like vomiting.

> I took mineral oil or milk of magnesia and it may help the next day. I don't start eating until everybody is in bed. I can't start when everybody is up looking at me because I know it's wrong. My father will yell and then my mother, so I can't eat when they are around. He tells me to go to bed or he just looks at me and mutters under his breath. He mutters that he wants to get rid of me or that I should be dead or something like that, that I am just no good or worthless. Sometimes he tells me that he wishes I would just go to bed and not wake up. My brothers say the same thing and so does my mother. They all want me to die and sometimes I think it wouldn't be a bad idea. I don't know, I have so many things wrong with me. I am not normal like every other girl my age. They are so alive and I feel just like sitting all the time.
>
> Everyone is in bed about 12:30. I begin to eat around 1 o'clock until about 3. I don't eat fast. If I ate fast, I could eat about 2 tons of food. Then I get so sleepy I can't get out of my chair. I doze off and try to get up and go to the bathroom and fall asleep there for an hour and a half. I sit down and can't hold my head up any longer and stay there until someone comes after me. I fall asleep while urinating. Then I get up and it takes me very long to go to bed. I use dental floss, everything takes me so long and I feel miserable. I brush off my clothes and sometimes wash out my underwear. It is then about 6 in the morning. Sometimes my mother will come in and see me in the bathroom and she'll start yelling and I'll start crying. Then we sometimes have arguments there. Father sometimes would run in and strike me and I would cry. Sometimes to spite my parents I will sing or hum outside their door late at night, sometimes a love song or something like that.

She denies hallucinations or delusions but sometimes looks in the mirror and imagines talking to her old boyfriend and how they used to talk and he would kiss her. Or sometimes she imagines she is quarreling with someone: a boyfriend or her cousins. She refers to this as daydreaming.

There follows in Dr. Romano's notes a personal history: Father, 46, was from Lithuania, in US Army at 33. Mother was 43. They lived in a three-bedroom flat where she had her own bedroom. Male siblings were 17 and 13. She was "dissatisfied with home life." Born in East Boston, she thinks she was "normal as an infant, although constipated." Chief memory of dancing a lot. People in the park would watch, gather around and watch her dance. Kindergarten at 4, first grade at 5. Commercial course in high school, graduated at 16. Liked English, not much interest in commercial course, but very good at bookkeeping, shorthand and typing. Does not think she was a feeding problem as a child. Believes present illness began three years ago at 18. Worked in a store but quit when "man I worked for started making advances."

Was going with boyfriend she liked, but mother nagged her into going with older man. Started to overeat and gained to 138 pounds. Went on a diet that mother disapproved of. "I had more confidence in myself because I was determined to lose weight and I was happy over every pound I lost." Went down to 90, then 82, doctor put her in hospital. Began to gain weight, remained at 92 for about a year, "Sort of felt better when I was thinner." Afraid if she started eating a lot, "wouldn't be able to control myself. I either eat too much or I don't eat at all." Spoke of being a patient of Dr. Kaufman and Dr. Jessner in hospital but "saw Dr. K's assistant (Dr. Waller?) most of the time." "He was young, probably 20s, can't recall his name" (although she saw him from October 1938 to March 1939). Saw Dr. Deutsch "just once" (Associative Anamnesis, reproduced above).

> He didn't say very much, I thought he acted kind of queer. He just looked at me and would ask one question and then look at me for a long time, didn't say much and wrote but I don't know what he wrote down.
>
> They (Drs. Kaufman and Deutsch?) would keep asking me questions about sex and my childhood. And they always wanted to separate me from my mother because they said while I was with her I would never get cured because she is very anxious and quarrels and notices every little thing. If I say one word, she'll run at me and strike me and pinch me and do everything. When I didn't gain weight, they [the doctors] thought probably if I went away from her I'd gain weight. They wanted me to go to relatives, but I quarreled with them and said I didn't want to. Then they wanted me to go to the State Hospital for observation and rest. I went but only stayed a day and a half. It was horrible, like a prison, I couldn't stand being there.

Her mother quarreled with the social worker and doctor at the hospital for sending her there and took her out. Patient said she stopped going to the BIH after that.

The patient returned to talking of her somatic symptoms: headaches, mucus in eyes, vaginal discharge, amenorrhea, and bloating of abdomen. At this point, Dr. Romano inquired about her bloated abdomen and whether there was a connection with bloating from eating and bloating from lack of menstruation. Romano noted "she remembered that when she had her menstrual period years ago her abdomen felt bloated. She was afraid that she might be pregnant. She was afraid because she didn't know very much." In the patient's words, "I was afraid because they had attempted intercourse with me." She said she had no physical signs of pregnancy to back up this fear. She said her bloating feeling from eating is as she imagines it would be if she were pregnant. She said she didn't think pregnancy would be a bloated feeling because "it's in the womb and not the stomach." As a little girl, she didn't know about babies. She remembered her mother's last pregnancy. She thought mother was just fat, and she doesn't like to be fat.

In spite of the trouble she has in the house and how unhappy she is there, she doesn't like to be alone with her daydreams. She feels as though she doesn't have a friend in the world. Eating makes her forget all these things. "I'll never be able to get married. I have so many things wrong with me."

In a first reference to mother's breast-feeding, Ms. B recalls seeing her breastfeed her younger brother but does not remember any feelings she had at the time. She denies envy of his place at mother's breast.

At the end of this session, Dr. Romano met again with Ms. B's mother. I note that her story is much the same as previously, with description of her daughter's unusual sleep pattern, disturbing bathroom habits, her sluggishness to take responsibility, sometimes "needing to force her." Ms. B again recounted the compulsive behavior of washing herself and shaking her clothes many times before dressing. She had recently begun hanging her clothes in mother's closet because she said her own "was too dusty." She described how doctors at the hospital had advised mother to give her daughter "her own way," which Ms. B says she did for two years, but mother didn't comply "for fear of spoiling me." She said father, "a sick man who only tries to make a living," was disgusted with her. Mother said her daughter didn't like Dr. K[aufman] because he asked her if she were jealous of her parents. She thought this was a silly thing to ask. She also said her daughter told her she was embarrassed when another doctor asked her if she didn't like the young doctor (Dr. Waller) who was handling her case. The patient told mother she "hoped he (the doctor) wasn't married." Mother recounted how her daughter went to a dance with a boyfriend and he wrote that she was "full of fun and called her Miss Massachusetts." The interview by Dr. Romano ended with mother saying "sometimes I would like to kill her; she is spiteful. But she don't lie; that kid don't lie."

In a shorter interview, Dr. Romano saw the patient on October 9, 1941. There must have been some contact before that since notes indicate that "patient says that since she was last seen in June, she has been better sometimes, sometimes worse." Before this June appointment, mother had written to Dr. Romano, offering as usual to "provide some facts" about her daughter's (and her own) situation. She describes daughter's symptoms of eye trouble, her slowness in everything ("that must be due to underdevelopment of something unknown to me"), her strange sleep habits, going to bed late in the morning, sleeping late in the day, and missing her appointments. "She eats like a horse in the middle of the night and doesn't eat during the day."

"When she was 13 she slept with me." She describes how the patient would like to move to another flat "because she doesn't like the house we live in." Reference is made to the compulsive behavior of wrapping everything or wiping furniture and so on. She makes the observation that "her fingers and palms of her hands are yellow." "Daughter talks very sensibly and no outsider detects that there is anything wrong with her." Concluding her letter, she requests that she "would like very much for her (daughter) to be admitted to the hospital for observation," adding that "if she would soon have her periods most of her troubles and abnormalities would be erased." Finally, she writes, "I hope this letter has made a few points clearer for you."

What seems like a rebuttal of mother's letter to Dr. Romano, the patient wrote her own letter to him. She begins

> if you should find me dead sometime, I want you to know that I suddenly didn't get insane, it was all my mother's fault. For years she has been at my throat. She has maimed me, scarred me, bitten and pinched every part of my body. Besides these physical hurts, she has nagged and cursed me so much until I have become a nervous wreck and she has taken away from me the last spark of energy I had left. Because of her, I have become a chronically sick girl and there is nothing left for me to live for. My eyes are worn and weary from crying from morning to night and she has upset every function in my body. I guess from the time I was born she hated me, and during the short years of my life made it a point either to kill me or make me want to die.

In the interview of October 9, the patient recounted her sleep and dream behavior. She most often goes to bed around 7 a.m. and sleeps until 2 p.m. Occasionally she has repetitive nightmares in which men are trying to harm her, feeling hands on her legs, waist and breasts, never pleasurable and "never dreams of intercourse." In her fright, she will call out for "Ma" and then minimizes the dream.

When she wakens in the afternoon, she will eat if there is no argument. If there are arguments with mother, she cries, mother gets upset and runs out of house, and then "patient sits and cries all day and doesn't dress." If she does get dressed, she will leave the house and go to a café for coffee and pie. Returning home feeling hungry, sits down to eat a little, begins reading and then

> stuffs herself with candy, cake and everything under the sun, then stays up the rest of the day until very late reading. I sometimes feel as if I eat with no appetite at all. Afterwards I feel so sick I just want to die. I cry. My mother or I will kill myself by turning on the gas or just overeating and ruining my intestines and getting ulcers and everything.

At one point she said

> I am so disgusted when my mother quarrels with me and I can't stand it. Even if I just ask her a question, she'll flare up and gets peeved, then I'll ask in a louder voice and she'll yell at me. Sometimes she thinks I'm doing it just for spite and she'll tell me that's crazy. When my mother gets going, someday she'll murder me. I never saw another mother raise her hands against her daughter and try to tear her flesh. I had bad scars on my face for about 8 months and everyone would ask where I got them, and I would say it was an accident or something. Some days when she (mother) gets really mad she can't control herself. Lately it has been terrible. I get so exhausted from nerves. I cry all day and my eyes are swollen.

"I don't think my eating is so peculiar, I just do eat because I feel so disgusted. Sometimes I think I could stop overeating if mother would just treat me like a normal child." "I would feel better if only my mother wouldn't argue with me, if she would only give me a chance." Says she doesn't have this trouble in other people's homes.

While she has dates and goes to movies and such, mother tells her the boys are afraid to make love to her. She has no sexual experiences on these dates "or anyone else." She does not masturbate (except as a child) and feels she would get "no satisfaction from touching myself."

At the end of this interview, she again brought up the harrowing short stay at the State Hospital (perhaps expecting that Dr. Romano might refer her there again). However, he "decided to refer me to the MGH for further study, perhaps with intensive workup over two or three weeks, when there could be opportunity for therapy with a good psychiatric social worker." Patient accepted this suggestion but "felt mother should be given a talking to also." After this study, according to Dr. Romano, someone will explore the community possibilities for foster home placement. "In the interim, Dr. Friedgood is going to attempt to induce menstruation with endocrine therapy."

Mother's response to this recommendation was that patient would probably not be able to get ready in time for her appointment with Dr. Friedgood and made a variety of requests to alter the appointment at mother and daughter's convenience. She said she worried about her daughter's sanity but brought with her evidence that she was not crazy: honor roll certificates, good report cards, and schoolwork extolling her brilliance. She wept and asked about shock treatment "if it was the only chance not to lose her daughter." She also brought a love letter to her daughter from a boyfriend. Another letter, not so loving, was written by the patient, accusing her mother of blighting her life and hating her since birth. The letter refers to her constant weeping, trouble with her eyes, and damage done to "every portion of my body." While mother felt bad about this, she said that when she herself was sick, her daughter would be quite upset and very solicitous of mother's well-being. Mother concluded with crying, saying "the family situation is becoming intolerable." "I would like to know if you think marriage would cure my daughter."

On December 16, 1941, Dr. Romano presented the case to a seminar on anorexia nervosa at the Boston Psychoanalytic Institute (BPSI). His preparatory notes, presumably drawn from his interviews, seemed to "interpret" patient's remarks, not exactly as spoken by her in the interviews. As presented to the seminar, here are Romano's talking points:

1 Compulsive eating. She said she had to keep things away from her mind by eating.
2 Significance of drinking water?
3 Significance of heavy makeup?
4 Memory of brother's birth at patient's age 3. Ideas of replacing brother at mother's breast. Wish to run away with father.
5 At age 6, thought kissing responsible for pregnancy.
6 Slept with brother. Swiped food from icebox at night and shared with brother. Eating as causative factor in pregnancy?
7 Until age 11, spent each night in bed with mother and father, between them, to keep them apart?
8 Reciprocal threats with mother of suicide. Conscious death wishes for mother.
9 Motive for staying up at night to keep father and mother from having intercourse.
10 Nausea associated with fiancé's attempt to have intercourse with her.
11 Duration of compulsive traits of wiping eyes and brushing off chair.
12 Falling asleep in bathroom.
13 Later preoccupation with thoughts of intercourse and rape by every male, including younger brother and uncle.

N.B. Some of these issues may have derived from clinical visits for which records are not available.

The Seminar on Psychoanalytic Psychiatry at Boston Psychoanalytic Society (BPSI) December 16, 1941: Dr. Romano Presents Case

The meeting begins with a recap of the history by Dr. Romano:

> a 21-year-old girl suffering from alternating periods of anorexia and ravenous eating. Details about this patient can be found in a paper by Dr. Kaufman and Dr. Deutsch [Dr. Waller is omitted] in *Psychosomatic Medicine* and in Dr. Deutsch's paper on Associative Anamnesis [indicating Romano's familiarity with these detailed accounts]. There is a marked disturbance of the sleep cycle; she

> sleeps a good part of the day, is awake most of the night and does much of her eating during the course of the night. She has a mucus discharge from her eyes and irritates her conjunctiva by wiping off mucus. Much concerned about her nose, she irritates the skin of her nose before a mirror. Compulsive rituals continue with vigorous shaking out her clothes to do away with possible contamination. She is very aggressive against her mother, who herself is an unstable, over-solicitous person. Violent outbursts of rage occur against her mother in which she throws things at her. Most of her time is spent sitting by herself and reading cheap literature. Amenorrhea has continued for two years. She had two half-hearted love affairs without forming any warm attachment with concern about the impression she makes upon the boy, particularly whether she is too fat. She is now at Massachusetts Mental Health Center (MMHC) where she has shown but little change. During interviews, she showed no obvious emotional disturbance and her affective state was adequate to the situation. She at least superficially had a good relationship with the examiner and showed no delusional or mood disturbance.

After this brief summary by Romano, the senior psychoanalyst attendees at the seminar largely dominated the meeting, Dr. Felix Deutsch stating that the patient had a good superficial relationship to her therapist [Dr. Waller] but that psychotherapy had no effect, that she had a strongly ambivalent relationship to her mother, mentioning at one time that her mother was too good to her and at other times complaining bitterly about her. He mentioned the familial factor in that father himself had an eating problem and stopped eating when angry. One analyst questioned the validity of the diagnosis of anorexia because of the patient's tendency to overeat. Both Dr. Deutsch and Dr. Erich Lindemann stressed that alternating phases of not eating and overeating were characteristic for anorexia nervosa.

Seminar members then referred to their own clinical experiences with anorexia patients; the most elaborate was that of Dr. Helene Deutsch (later expanded in a publication by Dr. Paul Roazen [1981]). She describes the difficulty of working with the patient, the complex transference, the equating of eating ritual with masturbation conflict and the tendency of the patient to act out fantasies which she has "learned from the analyst." Emphasis is placed on the importance of letting the patient assume control, although there is "little therapeutic benefit." Fantasies of oral impregnation through intake of food are not seen as attempts at procreation but rather a "terrible aggression against her mother, directed against the mother's womb, then followed by bathroom ceremonials of vomiting to eliminate what she has eaten." Dr. Felix Deutsch adds that pregnancy fantasies occur in neuroses other than anorexia.

The seminar ends with a discussion, introduced by Romano, of the differences between Simmonds' disease and anorexia. Dr. Erich Lindemann emphasizes that the clinical picture of anorexia is that of starvation rather than dysfunction of the endocrine glands. He also draws differential distinctions between eating disorders of depression and schizophrenia. Helene Deutsch mentions the salience of forbidden ceremonials. Dr. Charles Brenner concludes the meeting with the remark that "diagnosis of anorexia nervosa in the clinic is usually made on the basis of typical ceremonials surrounding eating habits in an individual with a special personality structure and that it is not made by exclusion."

Later Encounters

Dr. Lipsitt's Consultation

I was a third-year psychiatric resident, on the consultation service of a major teaching hospital (BIH) in Boston, when called to the emergency room on October 11, 1961 to evaluate a 42-year-old female patient "behaving strangely." Lying on a stretcher, she was grimacing and untalkative, waving hands and arms in the air in constant writhing and stereotypical motion, appearing to intensify when spoken to, though without the waxy flexibility of typical catatonia. She would pucker her mouth in snout-like fashion and make gnashing movements of her jaw. Frequent belching was followed with her only words "Oh, God" and the appearance of some relief. Otherwise, she looked pale, had dry skin, was facially expressionless and irritable when addressed by staff, and had minimal verbal responsiveness. She experienced a grand mal seizure while I was writing my clinical note.

I was urged by a busy emergency room staff, not known for patience with mentally disturbed patients, and by the patient's insistent mother, to transfer her to the state psychiatric hospital, where she had been admitted just 3 months before, following an "almost identical history" (absent the grand mal seizure witnessed on this emergency visit) and visit to the hospital's emergency service.

On this occasion, when she had low blood pressure, rapid pulse, and suggestive neurologic signs, I felt that an organic source of her affliction could not be ruled out by the cursory examination in the emergency department, and I felt that transfer to the psychiatric state hospital was inappropriate. The supervising physician somewhat reluctantly agreed to my urging that the patient be admitted medically for fuller assessment. Since the hospital had no psychiatric inpatient service or "dedicated" psychiatric beds at the time, admission to a medical floor proved propitious.

On transfer to a medical bed, the patient experienced a massive hematemesis requiring emergency transfusion of 10 units of blood. Curiously, x-rays of the gastrointestinal tract were equivocal, although she was presumptively considered to have a peptic ulcer and treated conservatively with infusions of milk, saline drip and appropriate medication. Nor did her blood studies show significant findings other than low thyroid activity, which was treated appropriately with thyroid extract.

Once the patient was under medical supervision and management, I had time to review her considerable medical record with detailed accounts of previous clinic visits and hospital admissions. My eye was particularly drawn to mention of the early contact with Dr. Felix Deutsch in 1938.

This was of some considerable interest for me since, with my acquaintance with psychosomatic medicine, including Deutsch's prominent role in the development of that field, his name carried significant psychiatric cache. Well recognized in psychiatric and psychoanalytic circles to have written prominently about "the mysterious leap from the mind to the body" (Deutsch, 1959), he had a notable influence on psychosomatic medicine. He had been not only Freud's personal internist in Vienna but a fully trained psychoanalyst known for first introducing the expression "psychosomatic medicine" in the literature of the early 1920s.

By association, I was reminded of Freud's early case (1905) of Dora and Deutsch's later (1957) critique of Freud's account of the case in "A fragment of an analysis of hysteria." Deutsch revealed that, as a practicing physician, he had treated Dora for somatic symptoms when she was 42, the same age as Ms. B on my first encounter with her.

In some sense, I imagined that by my new acquaintance with "Deutsch's patient" I was experiencing a kind of parallel to the long-term reconsideration of the Dora case (Jennings, 1986). Freud's Dora case was the foundation of psychoanalysis with important and generally applicable discoveries about the "talking cure," transference and countertransference (which is very important in the treatment of anorexia). Furthermore, when Dora was 18 years old, like our current patient, she had complained to Freud of "disgust at food," interpreted by Freud as a "regression from adolescent sexuality to forbidden infantile wishes." He first thought that anorexia might be associated with trauma surrounding food and eating or sexual abuse but later adopted the idea that, like hysteria, it was "an effect of fantasies of childhood seduction." Importantly, and reiterated by almost every therapist of patients with anorexia, he warned against efforts to treat anorexia psychoanalytically since the urgency of life-threatening aspects of the disease called for immediate physical intervention (Sayers, 1988). Sayers notes that "Freud's theory that anorexia expresses fantasy of oral sex was subsequently developed by Waller, Kaufman & Deutsch" (Sayers, 1988, p. 362) (see section on Orality).

Although my residency responsibilities did not require following a patient after emergency consultation, it was my decision, with this introduction, to continue with her with considerable enthusiasm. In 1989, after more than 20 years seeing the patient, I had written briefly (Lipsitt, 1989) of her in the 50th anniversary issue of *Psychosomatic Medicine*, describing Deutsch's development of the associative anamnesis, demonstrated with his/my patient.

Ms. B's Hospital Course

Inquiry into events preceding the patient's admission to the hospital shed light on mother's reaction to the patient's illness. A police ambulance had brought the patient to the hospital at 3:15 a.m., after a tumultuous night of extreme physical complaints. Mother found her daughter in their kitchen about an hour earlier, screaming, holding her chest and appearing unable to talk. Earlier, around 10 p.m., the daughter complained of epigastric distress and was emitting retching sounds in the bathroom, which mother first ignored since this was a frequent event. Mother retired to bed but was awakened by agonizing cries from the kitchen. As she entered to investigate, the daughter fell, only to be caught by mother. A police ambulance was called by mother, and the patient was brought and admitted to hospital (BIH) on October 11, 1961.

For the first two days of hospitalization, she was in a semi-comatose state. Nurses' notes during that time recorded open masturbation, writhing movements looking like mild convulsions and abdominal movements "suggestive of the bearing down seen in women with labor pains." On the third day, she was more responsive, complaining of painful hemorrhoids and marked hunger. She cried and laughed alternately, appearing depressed but telling staff she felt good. Marked abdominal distention gradually subsided. She drank copious amounts of water, with frequent urination.

Throughout a 6-week hospital course, Ms. B was described as pleasant and cooperative, even helping nursing staff assist other patients. No further bizarre behavior was noted other than excessive fluid intake, frequent trips to the bathroom and an irregular sleep pattern.

While in hospital, she was seen for psychological testing on November 14 by psychologist Dr. Judith Singer to "distinguish between organicity and hysteria" in explaining some of her presenting symptoms. The patient was described as cooperative but behaving "in the manner of an innocent little girl" who was "most eager to cooperate." She "demonstrated a wish to be cared for by older people" and "a feeling of abandoning herself to helplessness." "She often gives up and regresses quickly to a helpless position even when she has the correct solution available." "Having knowledge of things threatens her defensive position, with relinquishing of all personal strivings in a masochistic way, surrendering to whatever the external world wishes to do to her rather than face the basic dilemmas of her existence." Associative material suggested a "serious problem with masturbation, accompanied by fantasies of being pregnant or having a fantasied penis."

No organicity was detected, but "what is so striking about her total record is that she is not structurally psychotic, but rather a flagrant primitive hysteric with an extreme amount of narcissism, who, during a regression, can *function* as a psychotic." She is "relatively brittle and can regress quickly under pressure." She "cannot leave those she is ambivalently tied to." On a TAT (Thematic Apperception Test) card, she sees herself as "needing to deny herself any adult feminine role." She

> describes the picture of a girl asking where babies come from. The mother tries to tell her but the little girl becomes unhappy; she is not happy about the facts of life. She is surprised and unhappy and is turning her face away because she is so ashamed and modest (the patient's narrative interpretation of the picture on the card).

The psychologist summarizes her report

> this is a woman of hysterical character structure with massive infantile and narcissistic features who certainly can be functionally psychotic in the way she must lead her life as a small, innocent child. Further significant is very heavy coloring of sadomasochistic perversion where she is likely to provoke attack, enjoy the results, and to feel completely unresponsible for what has taken place. The openness of the hysterical conflicts and yet the inflexibility of her defensive structure states what her history confirms that she is an extremely limited individual who essentially lives in a psychotic way. It is the extent of the narcissism and the extreme ego investment in being a little girl that indicates that any kind of psychotherapeutic venture would be doomed to failure.

Dr. Robert Eisendrath's Interview

Seven days later, on November 22 (about 1 month after hospitalization), the patient was interviewed by psychiatric resident Dr. Robert Eisendrath, as follows.

DR: I was wondering how things are going since you have been in the hospital.

PT: Sometimes I can't remember everything that happened in the past. I feel very, very tired. I walk around and everything. I hate to lie in bed because once I get in bed I could stay there all the time. I fall asleep and it is hard for me to get up, and so I just keep walking, and I force myself to get around. I am very fatigued all the time, no energy.

DR: How long have you been feeling so fatigued?

PT: For a number of years. I have been getting more tired and more tired all the time. I'll say for about 5 years, or more even, on and off.

DR: How have things been going at home?

PT: At home things are quiet now. My parents are very nervous, but their tempers are a little more subsided.

DR: I don't know very much about your parents, so you will have to…are they nervous people?

PT: Yes, always nervous. My father is always home now, and he gets on my mother's nerves. He watches me, and he watches my mother, and she becomes upset, and then she takes it out on me.

DR: Is your father retired?

PT: Ya.

DR: Has he been working up until recently?

PT: He worked up until he was 65. Now he is 68 approximately. I think he has been retired for a couple of years now.

DR: What kind of a person is he?

PT: Ordinarily he is a very mild person on the outside, but in the house he is entirely different. He has no other interest except to watch what I'm doing and to watch what my mother's doing. He finds fault with everything and everyone.

DR: Has it always been that way?

PT: When he worked, no. He was more occupied and so it wasn't so bad.

DR: What was he like when he worked?

PT: He would work and come home and eat his supper and talk to my mother. It was always my mother that was a little bit more nervous than he was when he worked, and she used to complain about me, and then he started shouting at me, and it was like that at home.

DR: Why would he shout at you?

PT: Because she would tell him that I'm making her upset and nervous. And he would see how nervous she was and it would make him upset. And she would tell him that it was my fault, that I was doing this to her, otherwise she wouldn't be so nervous. It was me that was doing all this to her, and it would make him angry with me.

DR: Did he always side with her?

PT: Ya.

DR: Never took your side?

PT: No.

DR: You were never a "daddy's girl," huh?

PT: No. (laughs)

DR: You weren't?

PT: No.

DR: How come?

PT: How come? In the first place, if he ever did side with me, the rare occasions when he did take my part, she would just take the life out of him. I mean she wouldn't talk with him for a week, she wouldn't sleep with him, and she would tell him that she was going to commit suicide. She wouldn't do a thing like that, but she would tell him that. She would make things so unbearable for him that he would never side with me again.

DR: Did this ever happen?

PT: What?
DR: That he sided with you.
PT: Well, a long time ago it happened on a few occasions.
DR: Do you remember any of them?
PT: No. I don't, but I remember what did happen after he did side with me.
DR: When was the last time he sided with you?
PT: Maybe about 8 years ago. More than that.
DR: Did he ever side with you on any important decisions in your life?
PT: Well, many years ago, when my mother wanted me to go to this older boyfriend, at the beginning he felt that this fellow was too old for me.
DR: Did you agree?
PT: Oh yes, I didn't want to go at all. This happened a long time ago.
DR: He was interested in your whole life?
PT: Oh, it is so long, it is such a long story.
DR: I'd like to hear about it. We have a lot of time to spend.
PT: I don't know where to start.
DR: I wondered about your father in the past.
PT: My father. When I was going to school he ignored me completely. I'll just tell you about my father. He always liked the boys, the two boys, because he felt sons, well he thought sons were an honor to him, and that a daughter…well…there was just something to marry her off as soon as possible, and it was the end of that.
DR: His own daughter?
PT: Ya. Even when my kid brother had a child. I'm still a little nervous.
DR: Take your time. The recorder makes you a little nervous, doesn't it? It is just easier than writing.
PT: Ya, I understand that, but still I can't help but be a little nervous. When my kid brother, when his wife was pregnant, and she happened to have a daughter that day, and they called up our house and informed us that she had had a daughter, well my father began to cry because he so wanted my brother to have a son. He was so upset by that that he began to cry that she had a daughter, not a son. He was always like that though.
DR: Why did he feel that way?
PT: Well, I guess in the old country where he came from, they thought that a son was like a king, and a girl was hardly anything at all.
DR: Did you feel that way?
PT: No, I didn't. In my opinion, we're all equal.
DR: You have two brothers. You are the only girl.
PT: Ya, two brothers.
DR: How old are they?
PT: One of them is 38 and the other is 34.
DR: He was pleased when they were born?
PT: Oh, yeah.

DR: Do you remember when they were born?

PT: Ya.

DR: Do you?

PT: Sure.

DR: Was it an exciting time at home?

PT: Yes, it was very exciting.

DR: Would you tell me a little about it?

PT: We had big parties for the two boys.

DR: You were how old when your first brother was born?

PT: I was four.

DR: You remember that?

PT: Oh, yeah.

DR: Yeah?

PT: Yes, I remember, I was so happy. I asked the doctor how he came along, this little baby. He said he brought him in a suitcase. I remember I was looking at him, and he would open one eye, and then open the other eye, and I was staring at him. I was excited too.

DR: Where did you think the baby had come from?

PT: I didn't know.

DR: What did you think?

PT: I didn't have any idea, so I asked my mother. My mother was sick of course so I didn't ask her.

DR: Sick?

PT: I mean she was in bed, so I asked the doctor, and he told me that he had brought the baby in a suitcase, in this little satchel.

DR: How long did you believe that?

PT: Well, not for very long (laughter).
D. Did you find out?

PT: I found out where babies really come from when I was about ten or eleven. There was a girl upstairs and she told me. And I was all upset by it when she told me. I was shocked.

DR: What did she tell you that shocked you so much?

PT: She told me the way babies are born, and when parents had intercourse together, and to me it was a terrible thing for a man and woman to have intercourse together was a terrible thing I felt then and so I was shocked. And I cried to myself and I was terribly unhappy after she had told me this.

DR: You hadn't known about this before?

PT: No.

DR: Didn't you notice a difference between girls and boys?

PT: Oh, yes.

DR: What did you think about it?

PT: I thought that a boy—I had a boyfriend then, too—I liked boys.

DR: What did you think about the difference in the way boys and girls were built?

PT: I thought boys were built that way, and girls were built the other way. I didn't…

DR: You were an observer, so you noticed there was a difference, but what were your thoughts? Do you remember anything about it? It was a big discovery. You know you thought it was a big discovery where babies come from.

PT: Ya.

DR: So it was probably a big discovery about the difference between men and women, boys and girls.

PT: Well, I don't know. I always knew that a boy was of another sex, and a girl was of another sex, and then when they get older they get married and they have children. But I didn't know then when I was under ten or so, but I still didn't know how children were exactly born.

DR: Didn't you have some ideas?

PT: I did know that you had to be married, but that's all.

DR: That's good. What did you think? Did you have any ideas that turned out later not to be right?

PT: No.

DR: You know when children don't really have the answers, they make up answers, just like the doctor made up the story about being in the satchel. Do you remember any of your thoughts about where babies might come from, because I am sure you had some. That's an important thing. You were there in the family and saw one brother born and then another brother born. How old were you when the second brother was born?

PT: I was eight.

DR: What did you think about that?

PT: I knew my mother was very fat and I knew he was in her stomach because afterwards her stomach went down. She had become very fat, I knew that, and then after that…but I didn't know why she was fat. After he was born, I knew that he had come from a part of her stomach, or her abdomen. I didn't know what had happened to make her so fat.

DR: What did you think?

PT: I didn't know exactly. Gee, I really didn't have any idea…whether it was from eating. I don't know. I am just taking a guess.

DR: Well what about that? Certainly a lot of children think that.

PT: Because she had become awfully fat, I know that. And her breasts were enlarged. Her stomach was so large, she had become very fat, and then after my brother was born, everything began to go down.

DR: What about the idea…that you had something to do with it?

PT: No, I really didn't think that it came from me because I knew you had to be married. A man or woman had to be married to have a child, that's what I thought. I didn't really think that it came from eating, but I knew she had gotten very fat. I didn't know, I can't tell really.

DR: Maybe kissing?

PT: No, I didn't think it came from kissing.

DR: What did you think about your parents? Did your parents sleep in the same bed?

PT: Ya.

DR: What did you think about this? Did you connect this in any way?

PT: I think I may have, yes. Something about sleeping in the same bed. I know a man and woman had to be married. And something about sleeping in the same bed, too.

DR: And having to do with eating something too?

PT: I'm not sure about the eating part, but I remember she got very fat. Drinking a lot of milk, or I don't know what, what it was.

DR: Sometimes children have the feeling that their parents swallow something special when they are married. Did you have any idea like that?

PT: No, no. I didn't have any of those ideas.

DR: How did you feel when your brothers were born?

PT: I was happy about it.

DR: Were you?

PT: Yes.

DR: Why?

PT: Well, I like babies, and they were so cute. They were awfully big babies, they weren't homely babies. They were too big—one weighed 12 and the other 11 ½. And so they were big babies, and they looked like babies. When a baby is very tiny, it hardly looks like anything. And they were born in the house too.

DR: Did you see them being born?

PT: I saw them after they were born, and I remember the older of the two brothers, after he was born. I remember the other one, too.

DR: Did you see them being born?

PT: No I didn't. I was asleep, but I saw them after I awakened. I was happy about it. I liked dolls and I liked babies too.

DR: You didn't know where the first one came from, but you began to know where the second one came from, right?

PT: I knew that he came out of my mother's abdomen, somewhere.

DR: Let me ask you a little bit about your early life. Do you remember anything about your early childhood at all?

PT: Yes, I do.

DR: I know in the past you have had some difficulty eating.

PT: Yes, this was when I was 18. I could eat but I didn't want to eat at that time because I was becoming awfully emotionally upset then with this boyfriend that I didn't want. I was going with him, sort of obeying my mother, and was going with him reluctantly. I was in love with someone else, a fellow more my age, and I was just in love with him, and he liked me too, and we were thinking about someday we would be married, after he finished college, and I would also be doing something.

My mother didn't approve of him. When she met this other fellow, the older fellow, she thought that he was very attractive and he was making a wonderful living, and he was very bright. And she thought the world of the older fellow, and so she began to tell me lies about the one I was in love with, and she would catch him and tell him lies about me. We began to quarrel and I soon stopped seeing him because I was angry with him all the while I was still in love with him. I was angry and stopped seeing him and began going with the other fellow that I didn't care for too much. Soon, after I got to know the other fellow better, I told my mother that I didn't want to see him anymore because he was not for me, so my mother used to quarrel with me and beat me and whatnot, and I got terribly upset and continued to go with this other fellow, and he wanted to marry me, and I would say no, "not yet, not yet." "I don't know if I will marry you." "I'm not sure I'm in love with you." He kept wanting to marry me, wanting to marry me, and soon he began to touch me all over, and I told him I would stop seeing him if he was going to continue this. He said, let's get married, I want to marry you, and I said no, not yet, not yet, because I was really beginning to hate him. Except he was very attractive and all that, he was very handsome and making a good living, and was very intelligent, bright, but there were other things about him that I couldn't stand. I still loved really the first boyfriend. At one time, he almost had intercourse with me, not quite, but he almost did and I almost let him too, and so I pushed him off just in time, and I told him that I didn't want to see him ever again, and after that I began to be obsessed because I thought I was dirty. Although nothing had really happened, I felt that even by his touching me I was dirty, I felt sort of dirty. My mother was cross with me here and there, and then she would tell my father that I upset her, and my father began to growl at me, and she would beat me. Then this fellow came back again about two weeks later and said let's continue again, I still want to marry you, I still love you. I went with him a little while longer and then I finally broke up with him for good. My mother was so upset. You know I was engaged to him and I gave back his engagement ring and everything he had given me to show him that I didn't want to see him ever again, this was the end. My mother was so upset with this that she didn't stop quarreling with me and she beat me, and I couldn't go out of the house. She would take my face and mark it all up and whatnot, and my body and mark it all up.

DR: How?

PT: She would scratch me, take a broom and whack me. She had a ferocious temper, just like a wild animal in those days. She's not like that now but at that time she was like that. So I had to stop seeing all my friends, I was so marked up and they would say what happened to you and I'd be ashamed to tell them that my mother did this.

DR: How did she mark up your body?

PT: With her hands. She would dig her nails into me and pinch me, just wanted to tear me apart, and so she just grabbed at my whole body.

DR: Did your clothes protect you?

PT: Well, she would hit me with a broom. One time, she took some dishes and threw them at me, and they broke and I got cuts on my body, it penetrated my clothes. She would tear the clothes right off me many times. I would be going out and she would get armed with something or other, just any old thing, and she would tear the clothes right off me. She would dread I was going out or something and she would run towards me, grab my clothes; she was very strong too.

DR: What did she…

PT: I used to get hysterical. These things would start in for no reason at all.

DR: It still makes you sad, huh?

PT: Well, when I think of it, yes, although I have been thinking of it lately. I try not to, but whenever I start talking or thinking about it, I still, you know, feel upset.

DR: Yes. (Pause) Were you angry at her?

PT: Of course I was, and I used to think why is it that she hates me so. Like, in school I wasn't a bad person. I wasn't mean to her. All my friends liked me, my teachers liked me, everybody else liked me, but I'd come home and it seemed as though my parents disliked me, and so it would make me very upset, and I would think is something wrong with me that they hate me so? Because all my girlfriends' parents loved them, and everybody I knew, their parents were not like that to them.

DR: Maybe you thought there was something about you that they didn't like?

PT: Yes, I thought is it me, what's wrong with me that they hate me so?

DR: What did you think it might be? Something to do with being a girl, maybe?

PT: Yes, maybe a small part.

DR: What else?

PT: My mother used to keep calling me a witch. She'd swear and use curse words with me and tell me that I was a devil and a witch and whatnot. And it made me feel as though I am a very horrible person, although I wasn't.

DR: What made you feel horrible?

PT: My parents acted towards me as though I were a terrible person.

DR: Did you have any ideas at the time what it might be that they didn't like about you? It had something to do with going out with boys, didn't it? Your mother was so angry because you didn't marry this boy.

PT: Yes, and I had a lot of other boyfriends too, and I was very bright in school. My two brothers were not as bright as I was in school. I don't mean to brag, but it just happens to be true. I didn't think I was bright, but my teachers kept telling me and my marks were always…I always came out either one of the highest or the highest in the class, and I would always be amazed because I expected to fail all the time.

DR: What happened to this boy? Did he get married?

PT: Yes, a few years later though.

DR: Same?

PT: No, someone else, and it was someone…I like him as a friend, but not as a husband. I was not in love with him, I mean not enough to marry him. In fact, I did like someone else very much. In fact I was secretly in love with someone else who really liked me, but I felt there was something wrong with me. My mother would beat me, and I was always crying and I was emotionally upset. And I would call him and say I can't see you tonight because I was ashamed to see him. I wanted to see him when I looked my best. I was afraid he wouldn't want to see me again. So I would tell him I couldn't see him. I kept breaking one date after another with him, because I wanted to look my best with the other one. I was afraid that he wouldn't want to see me anymore, and so I kept seeing this other one that I wasn't in love with, and I didn't care if he broke up with me or not, so I kept going with him. I used to confide in him and tell him my troubles and we got used to each other, but I felt with him that he was a very good friend of mine, almost like a good girlfriend, a very close girlfriend. Finally my mother began to mix in again and kept telling me to marry him, I suppose because she wanted to get rid of me or something. I did like him as a friend, I didn't hate him, and then he was in the Army, and he told me that if I didn't marry him, that he wouldn't have anyone to come home to, and he'd be so miserable. And he had me crying for him, too. I felt so bad all around that I finally wanted to marry him, although I wasn't too happy about it. I acted as though I was happy at the wedding, but I really wasn't. Finally, I had to divorce him about five years later.

DR: Why?

PT: Oh, it was everything. He was a mother's baby. I didn't love him in the first place, and when he came out of the Army he wanted someone else to get him a job. He wanted to go into business, and he didn't have any money of his own. His mother kept mixing in. I don't know, it was just a very unhappy situation all around.

DR: Your sexual relations must have been difficult then.

PT: My what?

DR: Your sexual relations.

PT: We hadn't had any at all, in the first place. When I first married him I was afraid to because I felt I didn't love him enough, so at the beginning I was afraid to do that. But afterwards, when I got more used to him and I thought maybe I'll try to make the best of this marriage.

And I liked having my own home. I liked that part of it. But I thought, oh, if I could only be in love with the man I married, I'd be so happy living in my own home and taking care of it, and so on, but we hardly had any sexual relations then because he couldn't have an erection at all. We really didn't have any real sexual relations.

DR: Let me ask you some questions now about the eating problems you had when you broke up with the first man. What is your diet today?

PT: Today? It is a great big one. I eat too much.

DR: Do you eat everything?

PT: Yes, everything they give me, but I am on an ulcerative (sic) diet.

DR: What is your diet?

PT: It contains mostly milk for the ulcer, and I can't have any meat or chicken or fish.

DR: Is that what the doctor said?

PT: Yes. At the beginning I could hardly have anything. At first, after the blood transfusions...intravenous...I could just have milk and medicine. Then it was milk and cream and medicine, then gradually milk, cream and a little ice cream. They kept adding to it and at this time it is milk, mashed potatoes, mild strained vegetables, no acids at all.

DR: What about before your ulcer, before you came to the hospital this time?

PT: For a couple of years I have been having terrible heartburn and sourness and I could hardly eat anything, just the easiest things that would go down would be milk or ice cream or sometimes eggs.

DR: Did you live pretty much on a milk, ice cream and egg diet?

PT: Ya, and maybe some light cereal. That was the only thing that would go down without having any distress, you know.

DR: How was your weight during this time?

PT: I became very thin at one time, and then I became very fat.

DR: Do you ever diet?

PT: No, I didn't exactly diet, but it was hard for me to eat. My mouth would water and I would want to eat when I saw everybody else eating something. It smelled good, my mouth would water and I would just take a taste. And after the taste, it would keep coming up on me and it would tend towards sour-ish.

DR: How long had this been going on? Eating eggs, milk and ice cream?

PT: A couple of years.

DR: Before that, did you eat normally?

PT: On the outside, I would eat normally, not so much in the house, because in the house I felt unhappish (sic), but when I was outside I would eat normally.

DR: When you are unhappy, what are you doing?

PT: In the house, very little. Sometimes I would eat a good meal...until two years ago.

DR: Tell me about the time 23 years ago.

PT: When I broke up with this boyfriend, the one who almost...I almost but not quite had sexual relations with...I began to feel I was bad and dirty, or something. And I began to wash myself over and over again, and for long periods of time. I knew this was abnormal, and yet I felt I was going out of my mind, because I knew it was abnormal but I had to do this, otherwise I felt dirty all over, everywhere. It wasn't just my hands, it was all over.

DR: Did you touch the penis of this man with your hands?

PT: No, I didn't touch him.

DR: Did he touch you?

PT: He touched me on my breasts. He wanted to touch me down in the vagina, but I didn't allow it. Once he touched me in the vagina, but I pushed him away. He would talk about all the sexual relations he had had in the past. He was a travelling salesman and made a good living of course. He would sell to stores. Still, he would tell me all about his former sexual relations and it made me disgusted and nauseated, especially when he would tell me about the abnormal things he did with other women in the past.

DR: Like what?

PT: And so that is one of the reasons I began to hate him.

DR: What were the abnormal things he talked about?

PT: It's terrible. He finally told me this, and after this I just couldn't stand him. Some woman or prostitute took his sexual organ and put it in her mouth. When he told me this, I just couldn't stand him after. He told me that once he and this boyfriend had a little contest with some prostitute or some woman down in the South, to see how many times they could have intercourse with this particular woman. He said that he beat them all, that he had intercourse with her 11 times all in one period of time. After he told me these things, I began to hate him so badly that I finally broke off for good.

DR: It was the story about putting his organ in the woman's mouth that was most disturbing, huh?

PT: Umm.

DR: Had you ever heard of this before?

PT: No.

DR: It was a new idea, was it?

PT: Yes, at that time.

DR: Had he ever tried to do that with you?

PT: No, but it made me think that after we were married, he might after a while want to do that.

DR: So you started washing at this time?

PT: Yes, kept washing, and then I allowed myself to get very fat because I was overeating. I was very unhappy and I would be eating all the time. When I was alone I would be looking at a magazine and eating and eating, a lot of sweets and fattening foods, so I began to gain a lot of weight. When I started to wash a great deal, I decided I was going to go on a diet too, to have a complete overhauling. I began to eat less and less. And then the doctor was giving me a lot of Benzedrine tablets too. My mother was very upset because I didn't tell her why I broke off with him. I was ashamed to tell her because she wouldn't listen to me anyway. I could never speak to her or ask her questions about anything because she would get so upset at the slightest thing, so I didn't tell her why I broke up with him. She was so upset because on the surface he looked like a wonderful person, like someone who everyone would be proud of. But I wasn't, I despised him. My mother was getting at me, and I was so upset that I could hardly eat anything, at home anyway, because my mother used to beat me, and always arguing, and I would be crying all the time, so it was difficult for me to eat in the first place. Then when I was washing and all, and I wanted to lose weight. Then I began to eat less and less.

DR: Why did you eat less and less?

PT: I wanted to lose weight. I was angry with my mother. I was angry at the boyfriend. At that time I was still going with him for a little while longer, but I decided I was going to break off with him for good. I had it in my mind and I finally did.

DR: Were you blue, very depressed at that time?

PT: I was terribly upset. I knew that.

DR: You just didn't feel like eating, or you were disgusted with food?

PT: It isn't that I didn't feel like eating. It was just that I was going to make a complete change, get rid of him. He used to take me to these places and we used to have big large dinners, and I didn't want to do anything he wanted me to do. From then on, I just finally broke off with him.

DR: So you were getting even with him by not eating?

PT: Ya. He really wanted to marry me, even though he told me all these things.

DR: He wanted to marry you and he wanted you to eat good meals?

PT: Ya. Eat a lot and keep at the weight I was. I wanted to go against him and my mother.

DR: I see. Did you lose a lot of weight?

PT: Yes, a good deal. I went all the way down...I was a skeleton. I didn't like the way I looked because I knew all this was abnormal. I knew it wasn't right but I kept doing this. I didn't know why I kept doing this, but I was terribly angry with him and my mother. I went all the way down to 82 pounds and looked just like a skeleton.

DR: Did you stop then?

PT: Yes, then I stopped.

DR: How did you stop?

PT: First of all, I was washing a lot too. And I thought I was going out of my mind, and then I came here to the hospital, and someone suggested I should go to a psychiatric hospital and see what they say. I went there and then started to eat again while I was there.

DR: In the hospital?

PT: Yes.

DR: Did your periods stop?

PT: I never had really normal periods.

DR: Oh, really? Would you tell me just a little bit about that? When did your periods first start?

PT: When I was about 16, between 15 and 16.

DR: You never had any periods before that?

PT: No, before that I had never had any periods. I know I was a little bit disturbed by that because my girlfriends had periods when they were 11 and it took me so long.

DR: What did you think?

PT: I didn't know what to think. My mother was upset too. She was wondering what was wrong. Some doctor took a metabolism test and said my metabolism was very low and maybe that was the reason. He didn't know what to do for it, but said it was low and that might be the reason.

DR: What did he do, did he give you anything?

PT: No, I don't think so. I don't recall that he gave me anything.

DR: Did they start then?

PT: No, they started when I was about 16. Then I had a few and they'd stop. And then I'd have a few more, then stop a few more months. When I went down to 82 pounds I think they stopped completely for a couple of years. Then I started to get a few more, then it would stop again and it was very irregular.

DR: Have they been irregular all along? What is the frequency?

PT: Sometimes I would get six periods during the year. Then I wouldn't have anything again for six months. Then I'd have another four maybe to a year, maybe six, then I didn't have any for about four years at all.

DR: When was this? This period when you were dieting?

PT: Yes, I didn't have any for a few years then.

DR: Some girls are glad to get rid of their periods. How did you feel about it? Did you feel sad or glad. How did you feel?

PT: At first maybe I felt glad about it, but then I began to feel very unhappy about it, very abnormal, as though I wasn't a woman. I felt, gosh, there must be something wrong with me, I'm not a man or a woman. I felt very unhappy. Just at the beginning I felt a little happy when I wasn't eating right. But afterward I began to feel very unhappy about it, as though something was wrong with me, I wasn't normal, I wasn't even a normal human being, neither a man nor a woman.

DR: When you lost all this weight, did your figure change?

PT: No, I don't recall any real changes. Of course, when I lost weight, I was just like a skeleton, but I regained it when I gained the weight back. I didn't see any change.

DR: Let me ask you a little bit about your childhood history, your early childhood history. I've noted down some things I want to be sure and cover. You were born when?

PT: What year? I'm an old bag. I was born August 22, 1919.

DR: Do you remember anything about your early childhood besides your brothers being born?

PT: Yes, my school days, and I…

DR: What about before school? Let me ask you. Did you wet your bed?

PT: When I was a baby, naturally.

DR: After you became toilet trained?

PT: No.

DR: Did you have any accidents?

PT: No.

DR: Did you have any fears or nightmares?

PT: I used to have a lot of dreams. My mother would tell me about witches and boogeymen, and all kinds of things to be afraid of, and to watch out for this and that. So I guess I would have dreams anyway.

DR: Did you have a lot of nightmares?

PT: Yes, about people chasing me. My mother used to tell me to keep away from strange men, that they would kidnap me, so I would dream that a man was chasing me because he wanted to kill me, or grab me and kill me or kidnap me, or something.

DR: What else?

PT: Mostly about that. Somebody would chase me and I could hardly run because my legs could hardly move in my dream, and I'd be screaming or yelling in my dream, and my voice didn't even come out, I remember. I couldn't even run, my legs or feet hardly moved.

DR: Did you bite your nails?

PT: A little bit, not too much.

DR: Did you have a lot of fears during the daytime?

PT: No.

DR: Did you have any difficulties, anything that was difficult for you?

PT: No, I don't recall too much difficulty. Sometimes on and off—oh yes, I remember my mother. We went to a park on the 4th of July and they began to shoot these fireworks and suddenly there was a great big fire in the park. Some of the fireworks went into the trees and it started a huge fire and everybody started to scream. I was in the carriage, I remember, with a net over me to protect me from flies and mosquitoes. Everyone began to scream so much that I began to cry and scream. And I was afraid of fireworks for a long, long time. I had that fire in my mind—always afraid of fireworks, up until about 16. I dreaded it.

DR: What changed it?

PT: It changed suddenly when I started to be in love with this boyfriend, and we began to go out on dates together. I had a date with him the 4th of July, and I knew I had to go because we arranged the date with some other couples, and I liked them all, and I liked this boyfriend in particular. In those days they used to throw fireworks in the street. Now they don't and so I walked through, holding his hand. Ever since then I was never afraid of fireworks.

DR: Where you a good eater when you were a child?

PT: Yes, I was a good eater.

DR: You didn't throw up or have diarrhea?

PT: No, I never had diarrhea…I was always constipated.

DR: Did you throw up much?

PT: No, but I was always constipated. I had trouble there.

DR: Why was that?

PT: I don't know.

DR: What about your school days? Did you have any food preferences? Was there any food you particularly liked or disliked?

PT: I began to dislike milk. Oh, yes, about throwing up. I once had milk in school and I didn't know what it was. The cream was on top and it wasn't homogenized or something. And maybe I wasn't feeling good that day. I started to throw up and I didn't stop that day in school. So I didn't have milk for four years. I couldn't. I refused to drink milk. I probably had milk in my food mixed up in it. But I couldn't drink plain milk after that.

DR: What changed that, that you got to like milk again?

PT: I don't know what changed it.

DR: Do you remember any other feelings about food, one way or another, liking some better than others or disliking any as much as you disliked milk? How old were you when this happened?

PT: With the milk? I was in the third grade, seven years old. This is unrelated to me, but I was going to ask you if that helps, because I have trouble with my breathing, too.

DR: Not very much. You were telling me that you didn't like milk for four years. But you got to like it again.

PT: Yes. Maybe the dentist told me I should drink milk for the teeth and everything. I had all kinds of childhood disease too. I had scarlet fever, this and that, and so everybody told me I should drink milk because milk is very important to the health and so I began to drink milk again.

DR: Any other foods?

PT: That I had adverse to? No, I had a good appetite otherwise.

DR: Were you an active child?

PT: Yes, I used to like to play with my friends. I had a lot of friends.

DR: Did you run a lot, and move a lot? Were you a nervous kid?

PT: No, I was not nervous, except sometimes I would have a fear of a certain teacher. I remember that when I was in fourth grade I was told that this teacher was very strict, and I was terribly afraid of her. They told me all kinds of stories about her...how mean she was, and how strict she was, and when I came into her room, and whenever she had oral recitations, she would call on someone to read. I was scared stiff and I would begin to stutter. If I would feel nervous inwardly, I would begin to stutter badly, and I couldn't say the word at all.

DR: You couldn't get the words out of your mouth?

PT: No. I knew them. I just couldn't get the words out of my mouth. She called on me to read, and I read a few words and then I stopped because I couldn't get that word out. I remember the word. It was Wednesday and I just couldn't get it out of my mouth, and she thought I just didn't know. So she told me the word, she said Wednesday, but I still couldn't repeat it. She said "Wednesday, can't you hear me."? I said, yes, I hear you, but I still couldn't repeat it. I became tongue-tied. And she began to shout at me. She said, "Are you being stubborn."? She didn't understand what was going on. I couldn't tell her that I was upset or nervous. And so she began to shout at me and said "I want to see you after school." I saw her after school and she opened up a book and asked me to read for her. Again, she thought maybe I couldn't read and so she opened up a book and I started to stutter again. I couldn't say the words. She shouted "What's the matter with you? What's the matter, tell me." I began to cry and while I was crying she opened up the book and told me to read, and after I had cried, I read the whole thing to her perfectly without stuttering at all.

DR: How do you account for that?

PT: I guess I got it all out of my system, all my fears and everything, by crying. And I just read the whole thing perfectly without stuttering. She couldn't imagine, and then I told her that I stuttered sometimes. And she called my mother to school. She talked to my mother. After a while she began to find out that I was very bright in school. At first she thought I was stupid because I would never raise my hand and I always hid behind the other person because I was afraid she'd call on me to read or something, and I was always afraid I was going to stutter. After she got to know me, she always gave me all kinds of tests and they always came out kind of high. And after a while I was on the first row, first seat because my marks were the highest in the class. She had me sing in front of the class. And she called the other teachers in and had me sing for them because my voice for an 8-year-old child was more developed than the other children. Then I was bright in everything too. At first I was scared, so I didn't want to answer.

DR: Any other experiences when you were a child?

PT: Yes, she sort of blamed it on my mother or something. At home, my parents found fault with me all the time, and my mother started to complain about me too. At the end, when we were about to go into the fifth grade, she said "oh, if I could only adopt you and have you for my own."

DR: What did you think of that?

PT: She made me feel very good about it, I thought that was very nice, if it were possible.

DR: Would you have liked to go away from home?

PT: Yes, actually, because at home it was quite miserable. My parents always found fault with me. Always criticizing, always looking for something to find fault with.

DR: What about you? How did you react about this? Did it make you angry at all?

PT: It made me feel there was something wrong with me. I knew there was something but I didn't know what. It made me feel everybody else was much better than I was.

DR: Did you get sick at all or have any troubles during those years?

PT: Physically or emotionally?

DR: Either.

PT: Not emotionally then. I did have these childhood illnesses, everything.

DR: Did your mother ever explain the facts of life to you at this time?

PT: Never. She never did that.

DR: How did you find out?

PT: I told you. When I was about 10 years old the girl upstairs told me. And the way she put it, it seemed so dirty to me. I was so shocked that my own parents could do such a thing. I felt very disturbed. I couldn't get over it for some time and then I got over it.

DR: You heard them in the bedroom and wondered what they were doing?

PT: No. All I heard was them talking, but I didn't suspect anything like that until she told me, and then I was shocked.

DR: Somewhere in the record I noticed that you stay up very late at night.

PT: Yes, I have been staying up lately. It started out that I couldn't go to bed after a quarrel.

DR: With whom?

PT: My parents and then I'd been thinking about the past, and what happened in the past, and it was so difficult for me to go to bed.

DR: What part of the past did you think about?

PT: Where I didn't listen to my parents, where I had followed my own mind, and to listen to myself. But I finally gave in to my parents, and that everything came out wrong in the end. And here I was an old maid and nowhere and sick and so forth. So, I'd be feeling sort of sorry for myself, which doesn't help, but I couldn't help it…I do feel sorry. And I'd stay up and try to keep my mind, to get my mind off myself, and I'd read magazines. And gradually the night would pass, and I'd go to bed very, very late. Sometimes it would come out in the morning. And I hadn't been feeling very well in the daytime either.

DR: Did that disturb your mother?

PT: She always thought there was something wrong with me, whether things were going right or not.

DR: Did your parents know you were staying up so late?

PT: Oh, yes.

DR: How did they know?

PT: My father would go to the bathroom during the night, so he saw I was still up.

DR: Did that annoy him?

PT: Well, it didn't keep him from falling to sleep.

DR: Did you want him to?

PT: No.

DR: Was there any noise that disturbed them?

PT: No, not at night. I wanted them to sleep.

DR: Was their door open or closed?

PT: They keep their door closed anyway.

DR: Why is that?

PT: I don't know. They always close their door. Sometimes they talk about many things before they go to bed. Sometimes they talk about me too, so they close the door. I don't want to hear anyway.

DR: What else? Why else do they close the door?

PT: I don't know. It is just that they always close the door.

DR: Do you close your door?

PT: Yes, when I go to bed I close it partly.

DR: Not all the way?

PT: No, partly.

DR: Why else might they close their door all the way?

PT: Well, it isn't closed tightly like this door. It is just partly open.

DR: Their door or your door?

PT: Well, their door. My door is a little more open than theirs. I don't know, that's not my concern anyway. I don't want to hear what they're talking about anyway. Because if I hear, it makes me upset, so I don't want to hear. As far as intercourse, I don't know if they can have any or not. I don't know what they do because that's not my business in the first place. I don't want to hear them talking about it most of all.

DR: Do they have intercourse?

PT: I don't know.

DR: What do you think?

PT: Well, I don't know how it is with my father at that age.

DR: Did you ever discuss it with them?

PT: Oh, no.

DR: Did you ever discuss sex at all?

PT: Oh no, never. In the past, if I ever asked my mother a question, she would get all upset.

DR: What kind of questions would you ask?

PT: When I was very young, well like if I went out with someone and finally he wanted to touch me, I would tell my mother I'd feel terrible about it, or I didn't want to go with him anymore. She'd become all upset and would start shouting and yelling and saying "don't bother me, I don't want to hear about it." It would end up in a terrible fight and I would be crying and hysterical.

DR: What was the fight about?

PT: I don't know. I just couldn't ask her any questions. She just didn't understand anything I asked her.

DR: Why did she get so angry?

PT: She always gets upset. She was always like that.

DR: So sex seemed to upset her, huh?

PT: Well, sex or anything at all concerning me.

DR: Did you ever talk to her about masturbation?

PT: When I was a child, this happened, but I didn't tell her.

DR: What happened?

PT: About masturbation? When I was about 6 years old, I was doing this but didn't tell her at all because I was ashamed. She never mentioned sex. If they would ever talk about sex—they did talk about sex occasionally, I remember—my father and her would go into a room and talk about it quietly so I would not hear. But I would hear, but they made me feel as though it was something to be ashamed of, even between a married man and woman. They made me feel as though it was a shameful, dirty thing, because he always talked pretty loudly. He thought I couldn't hear. He has a little trouble hearing, in one ear. He was wounded once and so he talked a little louder and I could hear everything.

DR: What was said?

PT: Something about sex. He would talk about it quietly so that I shouldn't hear, as though it was a shameful thing.

DR: (Interjected) What did he say?

PT: I don't know about this man, this woman is not married now and he takes this woman out to dinner, has sexual intercourse with her. He would talk behind the door. Even when I was in my twenties. I remember that he would still do this as though it was a terribly shameful thing. Even after I was married, he would still talk to her quietly, although I heard everything he said, because he talked pretty loud and my hearing was good. I couldn't help but hear.

DR: So you didn't ever tell them about masturbating?

PT: No, no never.

DR: Did you masturbate very much?

PT: Well, then I began to feel very ashamed of it.

DR: When you were six?

PT: No, when I was about 7 or 8, I began to feel ashamed of it.

DR: How about later in your life?

PT: About masturbation? Maybe once in a while. It might have happened about once in six months or so, when I was still a child, once in a great, great while.

DR: Are you still ashamed about it?

PT: Well, I don't know what to think about it now. I really have no ideas on it now.

DR: Do you remember what you used to think about when you masturbated?

PT: When I was very young, about six, I thought it was a very comfortable feeling. When I was 9 or 10, once in a great while I would do that, but rarely. After that I would be ashamed that I had done it.

DR: What did you think about when you were doing it?

PT: I thought about it then in connection with a boy. I was ashamed and then I wouldn't do it for a long, long, long time.

DR: Did your brothers discuss sex?

PT: No, I never discussed sex with them, although when my kid brother was about 5, I had to sleep with my older brother until I got my own bedroom, until we moved and I got my own bedroom. And he used to want to touch me and I used to fight with him.

DR: He wanted to touch you?

PT: When he thought I was asleep, he wanted to touch me.

DR: Where?

PT: In the female sexual organs, and I would fight with him and tell him I didn't want to sleep with him, but I had to sleep with him until we moved. So I always had to be on the alert watching him.

DR: Did you know the births of your brothers?

PT: Oh, sure.

DR: Do you remember it?

PT: It was just a very happy time.

DR: Did you see the circumcision?

PT: Oh, no, I didn't see that.

DR: You didn't? How come?

PT: I don't know. I guess my mother didn't let me in the room or something.

DR: Do you know how it was done?

PT: I don't know how it was done.

DR: You didn't see it then?

PT: No, my mother wouldn't allow me to.

DR: How old were you when you got married?

PT: 25.

DR: How old were you when you were separated or divorced?

PT: I was married to him actually for five years.

DR: You were about 30. You are 43 now?

PT: 42.

DR: What has been going on for the past 15 years? Have you been working at all?

PT: A little bit, off and on.

DR: What kind of jobs?

PT: Clerical. Shorthand, typing, filing. And I worked at the Watertown Arsenal. I was an inspector for a while and connected with clerical work.

DR: Did you work most of the time or not work most of the time?

PT: I think I've not worked most of the time.

DR: Why?

PT: I don't know whether I didn't feel well. I'd begin to work and then I had to stop because we were fighting all the time. I'd have to come to work late. I had to stay up until very late because I'd come home to eat my supper and our fight would start and I'd have to wait until about one o'clock to eat and be crying all night long. We could be fighting, fighting, fighting and I'd be crying, crying, crying and I couldn't eat because I was so upset. My mother used to hit me too physically.

DR: What were you fighting about?

PT: The minute I'd come in the house, my mother would start fighting.

DR: You sound as though you have nothing to do with any of these, as though she just picks on you. Do you ever pick fights with her?

PT: I know what you mean. I didn't want to start a fight intentionally. I just wanted her to lay off me.

DR: Were you fighting with her before you got your ulcer pain?

PT: You mean just recently? No, we haven't fought for a long time.

DR: She's calmed down a lot?

PT: Ya, and then I ignore them too a great deal.

DR: When did you first begin to have your ulcer symptom, the pain in your abdomen?

PT: Mostly it was nausea and gas pains on top, and sourness and bitterness.

DR: Have you ever had periods of being dizzy or feeling weak and then feeling better by taking orange juice or milk or something like that? Have you ever felt weak or dizzy in the last few years?

PT: Yes, especially when I first get up, it is very difficult.

DR: In the morning? What do you do?

PT: I have to drink a lot of orange juice and then coffee. And I begin to take those tablets, no-doze awakeners. And at some periods of my life, the doctor gave me Dexedrine to wake me up. And I was so tired that I just can't wake up.

DR: Have you ever felt confused when you wake up?

PT: No, not confused.

DR: Have you ever felt confused or weak during the day?

PT: Well, not confused, just weak.

DR: Dizzy during the day?

PT: Mostly weak and fatigued and groggy, and I can hardly move sometimes. But I don't say it's confused because I know what's going on all the time. Only those two times when I became unconscious, of course.

DR: Had you ever become close to being unconscious before?

PT: Well, I fainted away a few times from the pain. I had very bad hemorrhoids and I fainted a few times from that.

DR: What are you doing currently besides being in the hospital? You're living at home?

PT: Ya, and I'm not working at all.

DR: Things are going better at home?

PT: Well, they've just quieted down, because I'm not very happy. I'm not terribly upset, but I'm unhappy too because my life is just going away and nothing is being accomplished. I have been sick and unable to eat, and I feel so weak and tired. Terribly weak and tired. Even though years ago when I used to go out on the street, I began to feel better after a while, seeing other people. Now, in the past couple of years, even when I go out in the street, I feel so weak and tired, I could hardly do anything and I'm really interested in doing something and I just can't do it.

DR: How are your periods now?

PT: I haven't had a period for a year and a half.

DR: Our time is up for today. Thank you very much.

PT: Thank you.

DR: I'll talk to you again before you leave the hospital.

PT: OK and thank you very much.

Ms. B's Hospital Discharge

The patient was discharged 6 weeks after admission to continue in recommended follow-up in outpatient psychiatry clinic. She was seen there by psychiatrist/psychoanalyst Dr. S (no notes available). Shortly after this arrangement, mother sent a lengthy typewritten letter to Dr. S

> "to thank you and all the other doctors who are taking such an interest in my daughter's case for the past several weeks. Because I want or must tell you more about my daughter, especially her habits at home, or in her case, her way of life while living in our house. That is the reason for this note.

Her abnormal way of life is, more than likely, due to her puzzling glandular condition which has existed for close to thirty years. When she is at home with us, she doesn't eat, she doesn't get dressed. She does not go to sleep for 2 or 3 nights at a time. She doesn't go out and has absolutely no will-power at all. She argues with me constantly about nothing at all, especially if I tell her to get dressed or even to eat. Any normal order at all brings on an argument that can be heard for streets away.

There is only one solution. She needs supervision and has to be 'ordered' around by routine method such as a nursing home. In my house, she will never (and I am sincere about this, from past experience) eat at all, leave alone adhere to a diet which you may give. Neither will she take medication of any kind. She will never take medicines by herself and if I have to remind her, then it is definite, because she never listens to me.

Therefore for [her] sake and yours and all the doctors who have tried so hard to help her while at your hospital, I sincerely hope that you will recommend that she go to a nursing home where she will get help and there she will take their 'orders' whereas at home she will go back to the same abnormal routine. I also want to say that both my husband and myself are sick and worn out from her troubles.

Again I want to thank you all for your constant trying to help [her].

Sincerely yours,

Mrs. B

P.S. [She] told me herself that because she knows she cannot get along with me at home, she is afraid that she might collapse again. She also told the social worker that she would like to be sent to a nursing home. The fact that she likes people is very helpful."

Following discharge from the hospital, arrangements were made for the patient to be transferred to a Recuperative Center. The following letter came from mother after the patient returned home. On February 5, 1962, one month and eight days after discharge, the following typewritten letter was sent to me. I had been seeing her daughter since her emergency admission on October 11, 1961.

She begins in a complimentary tone: "I want to thank you very much for the interest you are taking in my daughter's case." Many times she mentions that "she never had a doctor who takes as much interest in her as you do, and such sincere interest."

She immediately explains that she had to take her daughter home "because she had a very bad cold, but now she is feeling much better." She explains how she had put a $10 deposit with a widow on a room close to where they lived. "I don't know, if and when [she] moves there, the woman will be able to stand her." She describes the annoying habits of nose-blowing, throat-clearing, and "other abnormalities." "Even in the

Recuperative Center (RC), women in the room with her couldn't stand her noises, her habits, her compulsions., wrapping everything in bundles (toothbrushes, combs, clothes, everything)."

> I can't begin to tell you my feelings about her abnormal habits. At the RC, I myself was so ashamed of this that if I could have done a disappearing act when getting ready to take her out, I would have.

Now at home,

> "she is back to her former habits. She doesn't eat, she goes to sleep in the morning, never keeps appointments, doesn't get dressed...and I could go on and on.
>
> She tells me she would like to move as it isn't good for her to live with us, but then does nothing about it.
>
> It's the same with appointments. She seems to find excuses for everything. It's as though she can't get herself to do anything, yet under supervision in a 'home' or 'institution' of some kind, she 'obeys' orders almost perfectly. She doesn't have the push to do anything at all. She knows what is best for her, yet there is something lacking somewhere in her that doesn't allow her to do it.
>
> What can we do about all this? This condition has existed for years and both my life and my husband's are ruined on account of this girl, her abnormal actions in her life.
>
> She knows that she needs to go to the dentist, that she needs to see a doctor about her nose, and she knows that the ulcer that she has is due to neglect and aggravation, and still in spite of her knowing it all, she can't seem to get medical care and keep her outpatient appointments [This is while her daughter was actually seeing me in the clinic].
>
> It surely is a sad case. A one-room apartment would be a good idea for her, where she would have complete responsibility. Yet, we can't seem to get anywhere with her. I am all out of strength. What can you suggest? If you would like to see me and talk things over with me, I would appreciate it very much [Her wish to "steal" from her daughter's appointments?—author].
>
> Sincerely,
> Mrs. B"

References

Cobb, S., & Reid, J. (1950). *Emotions and Clinical Medicine*. New York: W.W. Norton & Company.

Deutsch, F. (1939). The associative anamnesis. *Psychoanalytic Quarterly*, 8, 354–381.
Deutsch, F. (1957). A footnote to Freud's "Fragment of an analysis of a case of hysteria". *Psychoanalytic Quarterly*, 26(2), 159–167.
Deutsch, F. (Ed.) (1959). *On the Mysterious Leap from the Mind to the Body: A Workshop Study on the Theory of Conversion*. New York: International Universities Press.
Fischer, N. (1989). Anorexia nervosa and unresolved rapprochement conflicts. A case study. *International Journal of Psychanalysis*, 70(Pt. 1), 41–54.
Freud, S. (1905). Fragment of an analysis of a case of hysteria. *Standard Edition*, 7, 1–122.
Jennings, J.J. (1986). The revival of "Dora": advances in psychoanalytic theory and technique. *Journal of the American Psychoanalytic Association*, 34(3), 607–635.
Lipsitt, D.R. (1989). Anorexia nervosa, Felix Deutsch, and the associative anamnesis: a psychosomatic kaleidoscope. *Psychosomatic Medicine*, 51, 597–601.
Lipsitt, D.R. (2017). *Foundations of Consultation-Liaison Psychiatry: The Bumpy Road to Specialization*. New York: Routledge.
Lipsitt, D.R. (2020). The brothers Gregg and general hospital psychiatry. *General Hospital Psychiatry*, 69, 117–118.
Phipps Psychiatric Clinic. (1966). *Learning about the Patient's Attitudes. Teaching Guide for Psychiatry Residents (After Adolf Meyer). Unsigned*. Baltimore, MD: Johns Hopkins Press.
Rahman, L., Richardson H.B., & Ripley, H.S. (1939). Anorexia nervosa and psychiatric observations. *Psychosomatic Medicine*, 1(3), 335–365.
Roazen, P. (1981). Anorexia nervosa: Helene Deutsch, M.D. *Bulletin of the Menninger Clinic*, 45(6),499–501.
Sayers, J. (1988). Anorexia, psychoanalysis, and feminism: fantasy and reality. *Journal of Adolescence*, 11(4), 361–371.
Waller, J.V., Kaufman, M.R., & Deutsch, F. (1940). Anorexia nervosa: a psychosomatic entity. *Psychosomatic Medicine*, 2, 3–16.
White, B.V. (1984). *Stanley Cobb: A Builder of the Modern Neurosciences*. Charlottesville: University of Virginia Press.

5 My Sessions with Ms. B

After the patient's hospitalization, I began seeing her on approximately a monthly basis since her early experiences and notations of previous doctors made it unlikely that a more deliberate therapeutic effort would be fruitful.

Integration Clinic

I saw Ms. B not in the psychiatry department but in the medical outpatient space that housed 45 medical and surgical clinics. After a brief exploratory study, I had found that patients referred to psychiatry from these other clinics rarely kept appointments or, if they did, were often considered after assessment "unsuitable for psychotherapy." Therefore, I chose to see these patients in their "home territory" and established the Integration Clinic (Lipsitt, 1964), where patients with extensive clinic visits could be seen for half-hour monthly visits and where psychiatric consultation could be readily accessible to physicians in other clinics. Most referred patients never questioned whether the clinic was psychiatric or "mental health" or even whether I was a psychiatrist. They usually came fairly faithfully to discuss their somatic complaints, leading hopefully to psychological awareness in the patients. In spite of mother's assertion that her daughter never kept appointments, she was fairly reliable in her half-hour visits.

As expected, many sessions were filled by Ms. B with a litany of somatic complaints and furor over her relationship with mother. Vital signs, including weight, were recorded on each visit by the nurse, and weight remained fairly stable around 128 for the next 3 years.

My early note in the medical chart was largely to acquaint physicians she would likely be seeing in other clinics with a summary of the patient's history. I wrote:

> This patient has long been known to the hospital, having been admitted most recently for convulsions of unknown etiology and massive hematemesis…I have known her since this admission and have

DOI: 10.4324/9781003208693-5

> followed her sporadically since that time. She has a long-standing psychiatric illness diagnosed many years ago as anorexia nervosa and her psychiatric condition is appreciably unchanged. She continues in a very hostile dependent relationship with her emotionally disturbed mother, and any attempt to disrupt this relationship has always met with serious obstacles and problems. I would strongly caution other physicians who might come in contact with this patient against initiating a process which might have as its goal the separation of mother and daughter. The only way this is likely to come about is if the patient initiates it herself and this is highly unlikely.
>
> The patient lives on a most peculiar diet of milk and ice cream and vitamin pills. When she is feeling ill, her complaints are often in a kind of 'pregnancy language,' describing herself as feeling she is 'carrying' too much, with episodes of nausea, bloating and severe constipation. She clearly recognizes the reality of the situation, knows she is not pregnant, but sometimes reacts mentally and physically as though she were. She has a long story of endocrine irregularities and erratic periods. She has been on thyroid extract somewhat episodically for many years, sometimes with lapses for long periods of time.
>
> Patient's mother is quite manipulative and frequently attempts to deal directly with doctors without first discussing with the patient. I have found it more suitable to avoid as much contact with the mother as possible and to deal directly with the patient in setting up appointments, giving prescriptions and so forth. Patient is fairly intelligent and is capable of demonstrating sound judgment on occasion. Very frequently mother forces her to lapse back into a regressed child-like state by taking over everything for her.

I added that "I would appreciate being notified whenever this patient is seen in outpatient clinics or admitted to the hospital."

Two years after we had begun, a note appeared in her medical record from Endocrinology Clinic, where she had been prescribed 2 grams of thyroid. The physician's note, besides recording medical findings, stated "mother and daughter are filled with hatred for one another, presenting one with an insoluble problem." A postscript stated, "I think this is an insoluble problem that will drag its way on and on, or else radical surgery in the form of removal of the patient from the home situation represents a remotely possible 'solution.'"

After an Endocrinology Clinic visit, Ms. B came the same day to the Integration Clinic without an established appointment, apologizing for missing her assigned time the week prior because of "weakness." I wrote that "she looked better than she had in a long time, not so depressed, and not making demands to be admitted to the hospital. She complained of symptoms that sounded like hyperventilation, for which I prescribed the old remedy of paper-bag breathing. For her depression, I had given a prescription of prolixin, which she had stopped but asked to begin again. Since all notes of the Integration Clinic were available in the medical record for all other clinic physicians to observe, I added emphatically once again a *nota bene* to be seen by them:

> I cannot stress too strongly how important it is to not get involved in trying to separate this girl from her mother, although it is admittedly tempting. This situation has existed since the patient was 19 and many, many attempts have been made to effect the separation, all to no avail. The only way it is likely to occur is if the patient does it herself or if natural causes bring it about.

She complained of "a feeling of fullness in her belly, nausea, stomach distress, and constipation. I wrote that

> pregnancy fantasies are still in evidence, although patient is capable of reality testing to know that this could not be possible. Her periods had returned regularly in past months. She continues on her ulcer diet, drinking milk and says 'I don't know how I gain weight on this diet.' (She remained around 128 pounds.)

Ms. B kept her appointment about one month later, complaining of "heaviness in the abdomen" and that she had been having fights with her father. "He scares me." Again, she expressed interest in coming into the hospital "for tests" and to "rest a while and get my strength back." She said she was too weak to keep her clinic appointments. I suggested that she take a cab or have her brother bring her. I also suggested that she should have a complete physical examination since she had not had one since her last admission. A medical clinic appointment was made, to be followed with another visit with me after her exam. I prescribed prolixin 1 mg daily to reduce anxiety and depression.

Medical visit was made 3 weeks later, focusing rather more on her psychiatric than medical history since hospitalization, again with complaints of epigastric distress, nausea and bloating. A systems review was recorded as negative, although the patient reported some sporadic rectal bleeding. (There is no record that this was pursued; it was probably assessed as hemorrhoidal bleeding. She was essentially "referred back to Integration Clinic" without a thorough examination.)

In the Integration Clinic, she complained that she thought the medical exam was not adequate, claiming her blood pressure had not been taken (although it was recorded). She reported that she had mild pretibial edema. "It appears to me," I wrote, "that patient's protesting her care was a way of seeking hospitalization to escape her home situation." Wish for hospitalization was probably prompted more by mother than the patient herself. Mother agitates a great deal, claiming social workers think her daughter belongs in the hospital. I had told her that I didn't feel there was any indication for hospitalization at the time, that she should continue her 'ulcer diet' for epigastric distress started during her hospital stay although a GI (gastrointestinal) series in July 1962 revealed "no abnormalities."

For the next few years, Ms. B continued to attend medical and endocrinology clinics sporadically, interspersed with visits to the Integration Clinic. It is noteworthy that as her focus became increasingly somatic, reference to her psychiatric history disappeared from the medical records.

A brief Social Service note stated that contacts were being pursued with the Jewish Family and Children's Service, but no follow-up existed. The case was closed by the social worker, indicating that "Dr. Lipsitt would be following the case."

In the next few years, multiple admissions to the hospital's surgical service provided treatment of a chronic leg ulceration of questionable etiology. By this time, she was 55 and living in a nursing home. The note from her eighth hospital admission for a venous ulcer on her left leg made no mention of her psychiatric history. Physical examination "revealed a middle-aged, exophthalmic female in no distress. She weighed 114. The only positive finding was a 10 × 12 mm (leg) ulcer, noted to be dry and crusted." She was discharged as improved on antibiotics and instructions for "home care."

Three weeks later, she was in the Gynecology Clinic, complaining of bleeding from her left labia of 3 years' duration.

> No history of intercourse in past twenty years. Irregular menses all her life. At age 40, had thyroid replacement and periods were regular until 50, when she entered menopause. Examination revealed healing labia determined to be benign. No further recommendations.

Again, she was seen in the Endocrinology Clinic on January 27, 1962, missing an appointment with me "because of the flu." I asked that she call me when feeling better. In the meantime, she said mother had found and reserved a room for her with a woman (never consummated).

I continued to see her for the next several years without much variation from one visit to the next.

Nursing Home and Apartment Visits

When, after 8 years with Ms. B, I left Beth Israel Hospital (BIH) in 1969 to establish a psychiatry department at Mount Auburn Hospital, I discontinued seeing her in the Integration Clinic but kept in touch with her by telephone and infrequent visits to her domiciliary sites. I visited her in 1977, 1982, 1987 at the nursing home she entered in 1970 (2 years after mother's death) and her independent apartment in 1999. She resided in the nursing homes for about 17 years before moving to communal housing with a woman she had known in the nursing home.

My visits were all announced in advance, and I brought her gifts of candy on each occasion. After cordial greetings, she would say "you haven't changed at all," reflecting her own sensitivity to the many physical changes she herself had undergone in intervening years. She was heavier and shorter than I had known her at the hospital, had a kyphotic hump, wore heavy orthopedic shoes that she explained were for serious leg bone problems, and apologized for the way she looked.

In my 1977 visit, she appeared younger than her 57 years. She had smooth skin and dyed black hair and was wearing silvery blue eyeglass frames more appropriate for a younger person. She explained that she had lived previously at a different nursing home "while mother was still alive" but did not like it and moved to this new one after mother's death at age 69. The "other place" was "less free," and she "likes this place better because it is more open, the other people are nicer," and she felt more free. She added that "certain aides or nurses make for a lot of aggravation not just for me but for others as well." She seemed comforted somewhat by the thought that she "was not alone, not different from the others," not singled out "as she used to be at home."

Conversation ensued with her usual focus on somatic symptoms: Synthroid makes her eyes less bulging; headaches are less severe than they used to be, especially when she got angry at mother or father; a recent admission to hospital for a varicose leg ulcer, slowly healing; cataract surgery, no tranquilizers or antidepressants and so on. She continued her visits to clinics at the BIH, where she was followed by a woman physician that she liked, but she no longer saw psychiatrists. Hypochondriacal preoccupations probably helped to repress and obscure conflictual issues of guilt, anger, shame and the like, as postulated by Freud, "put[ting] the most powerful obstacles in the way of recovery" through this compromised mental state (Freud, 1923, p. 27; Lipsitt, 1974).

Surprisingly, mother's death was hardly mentioned during this visit. She was not sure what mother died from, thought maybe some form of blood cancer. I was still at the BIH in 1968 and had talked with her five weeks after mother's death at that time. As though trying to find nice things to say about mother, she remarked, "even while she was very sick, she still did things for me…she came to the hospital to cut my toenails." Mention was made of how she had spoken recently to mother on the phone when she "sounded strong again, even yelled at me, but I felt happy because it was like her old self." Laughing, she said "it seemed like old times."

When I said it must have been hard for her to lose mother "even though she had trouble with her," she began crying and said "I was always very dependent on her, like a child, even though she probably made me dependent." When Ms. B visited mother in the hospital, "she (mother) was weak and fell on her bed." When she heard later that day that mother had died, she "got tight, panicky, with scared feeling in the stomach." At the funeral next day, "a cousin reminded me of all the boyfriends I used to have" (like being free to pursue boyfriends without mother's interference). She thought that "others at the funeral cried more than me; I kept it all in, but I cry when I am by myself." She mentioned seeing a social worker after mother's death and said he was helpful because she "needed someone." Mention was made of how she went into the Boston State Hospital when mother was sick and hospitalized because "I was hysterical at home with father." She said that if she had remained at home, she felt that she "would have had a very hard time, might even have gone psychotic" (fear of being alone with father?).

She referred to father's death eight months previously, how he had heart trouble but did not go to the doctor. He was found by Ms. B's brother in a copious pool of blood, allegedly from shaving (but I had wondered silently about the possibility of suicide after death of his wife). She went to his funeral and was upset, but "there is so much commotion at the nursing home" that she "doesn't have time to think about it."

Ms. B did not appear depressed or psychotic to me. She seemed to have made a fairly reasonable adaptation to the nursing home environment. No longer did she have the hand-washing compulsion, but a view of her bed area revealed her belongings all neatly packed in various containers. The bed was nearest the window as well as the bathroom. She claimed that, because others will yell at her if she takes too long, she did not use the shower. The room was shared with two other women: one her own age with epilepsy that she "gets along with" and an older woman who "seems to have a mental condition with ups and downs."

With mild evidence of pride, she explained that she had been elected to the home's Executive Committee and was chairman of the Nutrition Committee. As though possibly expecting the kind of negative responses she got from mother on her accomplishments, she said that one nursing home aide in particular "resents people who do things for themselves, or if they are smart."

Impressively, she had given up her "strange food habits and now eats regular meals with other residents of the home," explaining that "it is not possible to maintain the kinds of habits I had at home" because "everyone here does pretty much the same thing." She still watches TV until late bedtime "but gets up in time for breakfast."

Before father died, he and her two brothers would visit her occasionally and bring things she needed. Talking mostly about her younger brother, she seemed especially impressed that he had a 17-year-old daughter who was born with a neurological deficit. My impression was that she identified strongly with this girl, and much more is said of her in my later visit.

Her early acquaintance with Dr. Felix Deutsch was recalled but with little memory of his actual interview, only that "mother had me seen by him because she felt I had to cleanse myself because I was eating peculiarly and vomiting." Memory, she said, was not so good since "mother had me get ECT [electroconvulsive therapy] because I was depressed when the man I was going to marry was killed." (The matter of boyfriend, engagement, marriage, and fiery arguments with parents seemed pivotal in either the origin of her anorexia or fundamental in sustaining it and appears in some detail in every interview.)

Finally, in this visit, Ms. B eagerly described a stray cat she had adopted, enjoying caring and buying food for it and the like. (Increased reference to this "pet" that she adopted "as a kitten" follows in my later visits with the patient.)

My next visit with Ms. B was not until 5 years later, on December 29, 1982.

I arrived shortly after supper time in the home and was greeted cordially by Ms. B, seeming a bit uneasy at my presence this time. I wished her a happy new year and handed her a box of butterscotch, which she timidly accepted and placed on the table. Dressed in a housecoat, curtain drawn around her bed, she apologized for her "messiness." Again, she emphasized how I did not appear to have changed, reflectively referring to how she had gotten "much older, with orthopedic bone problems and back pain." She reminisced how, at high school graduation, she was praised by her teachers for "being a model of good posture, but now it is very different." The special shoes were in evidence, as was the copious "stuff" around her bed. Her hair appeared dyed and her skin seemed quite well preserved.

She was still attending BIH clinics for bone and endocrinological problems, complaining that she had "no specific doctor; they all rotate." She continues taking thyroid extract 0.15 mg, vitamin D and calcium. The ulcer of "many years ago" was mentioned, now remaining on a bland diet (there was a container of yogurt on her table). Because she "couldn't trust the nurse to do it right," she "takes care of all medical needs and dressings (for leg ulcer), putting on creams and lotions." She continued to eat at "regular times" in the dining hall, although "other women eat in their rooms."

There were now two roommates, one of whom would frequently interject a word or two into Ms. B's conversation, usually a reminder of something the patient was talking about or at times a comment about the patient's past, a detail the roommate had gleaned from the patient's conversations, raising questions about her father and his work. In spite of this intrusion, Ms. B, smiling, said they "get along well, with only occasional fights or arguments that aren't serious." When she said arguments occurred deciding who will get something, I said I guessed that was likely to happen in any close quarters. She retorted "it even happens in some people's homes with families."

In the midst of our conversation, a cat ran into the room, eliciting a joyful greeting by the patient. I said I recalled the cat from my last visit. The cat had wandered into the home "as a kitten about 7 years ago," she said. Ms. B "came to be in charge of the cat when certain staff members left." She and her two roommates chipped in to buy food for the cat; there were several dishes set on the floor "for different kinds of food." At times when her brother visited, he would bring food for the cat.

Returning to talk about her bone problem, she said that she should have done something about it 15 years or so ago but that she "got into fights with mother over hospital and doctor appointments." She seemed to pause as though not wanting to vilify mother and said rather unemotionally that she "didn't know why mother was the way she was," that she "loved my mother but hated how she treated me." Mother, she continued, "turned other people...especially brothers...away from me, telling people things about me that weren't true." Since the deaths of her parents, she said she "gets along much better with my two brothers, 4 and 8 ½ years younger." Father was recalled as having "died about 3 years ago" (although my recollection was that she had told me of his death during my visit 5 years previously). She elaborated more this time about his death, describing how the older brother had found father at home in the bathroom with "blood all over the wall and the floor." He had heart disease, she said, and should have gone to the hospital when he was having trouble breathing, but delayed (as she also frequently did).

The brother was "very close" to father and very upset at his death. Father was "very neat," she said, keeping everything organized in closets, ironing his own clothes (? like patient's compulsive behavior). He attended veterans' affairs (World War I), synagogue (he was religious), worked until 65 as a tailor, active until he died at age 84. Elaborating further about him, Ms. B spoke of how father "hated girls," felt "they were nothing," how he cried when one of his sons had two daughters, although he "got to feel a bit differently towards them as time went on, maybe even towards me." Reminded of brother's daughter with a neurological problem, she spoke of how that girl "had brain damage from birth, never able to walk or learn things." Parents could not find a doctor or hospital "that they could feel good about, having been told the daughter would outgrow it, but she never did." Ms. B said "the girl's parents now worried about what would happen to the girl if something should happen to them." (Identification with this impaired girl seemed clear, with thoughts of both her own parents gone, with her own bad luck, having been born a girl, helped too late or not at all, doctors not able to cure her and so on.)

As our meeting wound down, she asked me about my hospital job and family. Since I saw no objection in this kind of non-therapeutic setting, I responded to her questions about my children and I told her I had two sons and what they did (as her roommates uttered "oohs" and "aahs"). It was my feeling that perhaps I had erred, and I could not tell whether she was distressed by this revelation or whether she would feel I came to see her as "the girl in my family."

As the visit was coming to a close, I asked her whether she would be willing to sign permission for me to access her hospital records and to use that material for educational purposes. There was no hesitation and a roommate served as witness.

My impression from this visit was that the roommate who interjected herself in our conversation was like a mother surrogate but more benign than her real mother. Hypochondriacal (and organic) concerns continued along with thoughts that she "could have a stroke." The cat, adopted as a kitten, was treated like a baby and gave her much satisfaction and pleasure. She continued on the Governing Council and, given her chronic problems, had made a reasonable adaptation to nursing home life. With increased distance from the deaths of her parents, she was more able to speak of them without anger and perhaps even with a modicum of insight. Of note is the fact that in her older age, visits from father and brothers had not been uncommon (perhaps "detoxification" of the family constellation with mother gone).

My next visit was another five years later, in 1987. Ms. B had now resided in this nursing home for 16 or 17 years. I typically called ahead to tell staff to let Ms. B know I was coming. But when I arrived, she said she had not been told, was surprised and embarrassed and apologized for "not having dressed or fixed up." I handed her a box of candy and said I would wait until she had time to ready herself.

As I waited, two nurses (Karen and Linda) seemed interested and concerned about their patient and asked to talk with me. They said Ms. B was "a very nice person" and asked whether she "really had something serious or was she simply hypochondriacal." She "seems like she should be able to function better, live on her own, be more active" (the "missing parts" of maturity). On one occasion, they said, this question had been addressed to the patient and "she became unraveled and sick." (Author: penetrating hypochondriacal defenses often threatens patients with decompensation. See Lipsitt, 2001.) Linda said she had a good talking relationship with Ms. B. She said that they talked about the patient's mother and that Linda could understand "because I also have a crazy mother." She said she "loves Ms. B," although she sometimes gets angry at her; however, Ms. B "knows it does not mean our relationship is in danger or broken." Linda said Ms. B shared stories about her mother "but never spoke of father." They also talked about Ms. B's early relationships and romances. Ms. B told Linda she had been married and divorced and because her husband was in the Army, he had been sent to the Philippines while she returned to be with <u>his</u> mother. She told the nurses that she had spent little time with him and also that "a man had been killed in auto accident on his way to the wedding."

Linda and Karen explained how they each had "different styles" of caring for patients, Karen being more of the disciplinarian, always telling Ms. B that "it has nothing to do with her, just this is the way I am with all patients." Linda said she "would scream if I see another old person, but I really feel close to Ms. B and like her." Both nurses felt that Ms. B "complained more than she had to" of osteoporosis, bone problems, arthritis, burning feet, and so on. Although

> her behavior is much as it has always been, she was now afraid that she may have cancer of the kidney, having been told by a doctor that she could have an obstruction from a tumor. She is always preoccupied with her body and discomfort.

Weekly visits (or more) to doctors are a common event. Ms. B eats with others and seems to maintain weight, they told me, although she is "picky" about food, her clothes and her room. She always takes long getting ready for the van to the hospital and "seems very obsessive and compulsive." Since she has no refrigerator, she keeps juice and some food in her room. Ms. B "gets upset with rules of a new administration, and if her pills are not given to her at exactly the right time." On one occasion, administration had threatened to discharge her from the home because of her demandingness, especially about pills. The nurses told me Ms. B was not on any antidepressants or tranquilizers, although she takes many other medicines.

Much to my surprise, I was told by the nurses that the "cat had to be killed" because "management didn't like having a sick cat in the home." They explained how upset Ms. B became, requiring Valium for a couple of days but "then adjusting to it."

Finally, Ms. B reemerged, Linda exclaiming "I thought you had eloped." In front of the patient, Linda said positive things about her and "I would like to take her home with me." Ms. B seemed pleasant and open with me, not reluctant to talk, as though picking up where we had left off five years previously. Typically, she went into great detail about physical problems, belly pain, concerns about questions of kidney disease, bloating "as though I am going to explode," heartburn, burning feet (needing 40 pairs of shoes), osteoporosis, constant constipation, loss of height by 3–4 inches, still a "night person" but sleeping pretty well. She takes lots of laxatives and was told by her doctor that her "rectum is very tight, that the opening is small, and that the doctor even had a hard time examining me." On the positive side, she had not been having trouble with her stomach ulcer. She had had a normal upper GI series and a barium enema that was painful and not too satisfactory.

In a description of an event of which I was not aware, she said that on a visit home some time ago, she got sick and had "been in a coma" for 2 days and "had a cardiac arrest." Admission to BIH was arranged but had no details about it. I asked whether she received all her care at BIH now. She had a woman doctor (Dr. V) that she liked. Once again, I asked whether she remembered Dr. Deutsch. She did and explained (again) how she had been taken to the clinic by her mother, thought "I was the first person with anorexia, although there are many people who have it now." I explained that it was a condition known for many years but that she was an early case in the 20th century.

This discussion seemed to trigger a spontaneous return to talking about the "terrible relationship" she had with mother, how

> there was a neighborhood boy I liked from the age of 12 and that mother also seemed to like until I was around 16 when he and I became more interested in each other, exchanged rings and talked about intentions to marry.

Mother "became furious, didn't want me to see him anymore." They eventually broke up. What happened to him?, I asked. She said she didn't know, although I thought (but didn't mention) that he had perhaps suicided. (This material about boyfriends, marriage, divorce, and so on has always been a large focus in her interviews and, with each telling, has always seemed quite muddled.)

> I continued to have boyfriends, was popular, smart, did well in school in a commercial course. But my parents never respected me because I was a girl. My father liked sons but he felt girls were of no use. I always felt there was something wrong with me. I couldn't understand how my own parents could hate me so much, especially my mother.

Father was an orthodox religious Jew who would take sons to temple and religious school.

After she broke up at age 18 with the boy she wanted to marry, her mother wanted her to go with a man 11 years older. It was during this time, she said, that she began to have "eating problems" and began to "eat a lot when he professed love for me." Although she "liked him as a friend," he "would get fresh with me sexually. Sex wasn't looked on with the freedom of today."

The "eating problem" caused her to eat a lot, gaining weight to 138 pounds. "Mother was very upset, didn't know why I did this." Then she began to lose weight and "just kept on going, pretending to be upset on the loss of each pound, but actually feeling very happy because it felt like getting back at mother." Dropping to 83 pounds, she was then hospitalized psychiatrically and encouraged to eat and gain weight again. This was the time she was seen by Dr. Deutsch and treated by Dr. Waller.

"I had a terrible relationship with my mother. She seemed like she wanted to take care of me, but then she wouldn't." On one occasion Ms. had

> met a young medical student from Virginia that I had taken a liking to. I arranged to meet him at the Metropolitan Theatre but when I asked her for taxi fare she refused to give it to me and there was no way for me to reach him waiting outside at the theatre. My mother attacked me physically, groping at my throat and tearing her fingernails into my face so that I was disfigured for a while, my eyelid drooped, and I had cuts over my lip and nose. The boy's aunt later called to say he felt stood up but I was afraid to say anything about what happened because I was afraid my mother would kill me.

Eventually, Ms. B did marry the "older man" (approved of by parents because he "made a good living") but "didn't really like him and divorced about 5 years later," returned to her parents' home, later "tried living on my own, but I was frightened thinking there were men peering in my window."

Once again, she mentioned how mother died of lymphoma around the time Ms. B entered the nursing home. Father died about 3 years ago of a heart attack. He had been brought by a brother to visit her in the nursing home from time to time (seldom mentioned). In association to this reference to parents, she said "I wouldn't care if I died, but I wouldn't kill myself." At that point, she teared up, was quiet for a few moments, then mentioned the cat "dying a couple of years ago." She spoke extensively about how smart the cat was and how it could let people know what it wanted, like opening the elevator door and so on. As she spoke of the cat, she began to brighten, describing how it would follow her around, sit next to her, how friendly it was. Almost in an explosive expression of feeling, she said "it was my baby." She said the administration was too strict and unfeeling.

When she mentioned the administration in the nursing home, I asked what her alternatives were, whether she thought she could live by herself. She said she couldn't do it, "especially after being in the nursing home for so many years." She added that she didn't want the nurses to know she had been in a psychiatric hospital. At times, "I thought I would go crazy with mother, couldn't understand her, always thought there was something wrong with me." I said that her mother was very disturbed, intending to relieve some of her own guilt.

My impression of this visit was that Ms. B appeared remarkably as she had in 1982, continuing to adapt to circumstances and even to mourn the losses of parents and pet cat. She appeared socially appropriate, asking about my family again. Linda was a concerned and supportive asset, while Karen may have been more of "another mother surrogate" (making patient feel much "at home"). The nurses appeared to have a desire for more communication and coordination of care. I explained that I would be glad to talk with those treating her but that I was not actually treating her myself at this point.

Ending the visit, I said I would see her again. When I asked about her concerns about kidney disease and fear of cancer and scheduled hospital appointments, she teared up a bit but quickly composed herself as I bid goodbye.

The next time I visited her, on January 9, 1999, she had left the nursing home and was living in a communal housing apartment in another town with a woman she had met in the nursing home. I had lost track of her since she left the nursing homes where she had resided for 29 years, but I was able to locate her in her new quarters by calling her brother for a phone number. My call to her elicited a more-or-less muted response (perhaps until she recognized me). My greeting and happy new year wishes and desire to visit then evoked the usual "the place is a mess" and "I've shrunk 9 inches." I simply assured her the house was not important, I would be coming to visit her.

In my visit, I noted that her home was an apartment in a large residential building that was part of a small housing community. On my arrival, the apartment door was open, and she said she was waiting for me, shook hands and said it was nice to see me. The whole building housed only 15 people, she said, much better than where she had been living (the nursing home). She was placed here by a social worker about 8 years ago during a hospitalization at the BIH. That hospitalization, she said, had been for "coma" and "cardiac arrest."

She wore a red blouse with a big bow at the neck, a kind of 1950s look, and the usual ugly black orthopedic shoes (Figure 5.1). She now used a four-pronged walker. Sitting side-by-side on a sofa with her companion (Figure 5.2), she smiled a lot, seemed happy, spoke of how well the two of them got along, although her roommate seemed to fulfill some of the nagging, pressured attitudes so familiar to the patient from her mother. The woman, Catholic (not Jewish), said "we get along pretty well, sometimes annoyed with one another, but we get over it." Many Jewish artifacts adorned the room, a Jewish calendar over the sofa, some religious items glued to the wall.

To the left was a compact kitchen with microwave and refrigerator covered with reminders of medical appointments, schedules, phone numbers and so on. Near the sofa was a large bin full of medicine bottles, tubes, salves and the like, many of which she no longer took (but did not discard). To the right of the sofa on a small table was a dish of M&Ms and mints, a clock that "spoke" the hour, and a telephone.

I had only a glimpse of the bedroom, which seemed, as it had in the nursing home, cluttered with boxes, a cane hanging on the doorknob and several bottles of laundry detergent on the floor. She retrieved family pictures from her bedroom to show me and asked whether I would like to see "pictures of me when I was younger." I was aware she wanted me to think of her "as she was." Family pictures mimicked familiar domestic scenes, with two brothers, one of mother and father standing with a

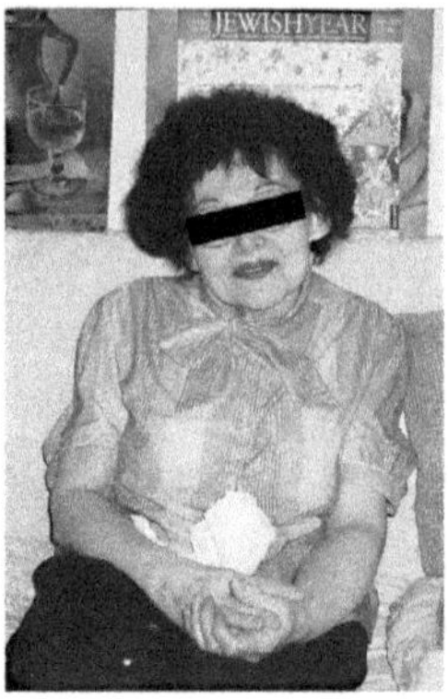

Figure 5.1 The patient.

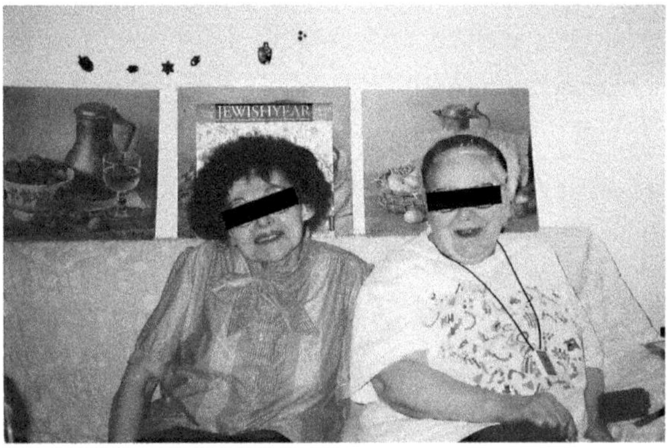

Figure 5.2 The patient and her companion in their apartment.

strikingly beautiful slim-waisted girl next to father who held her hand, brothers and wives next to mother, an idyllic image unlike any described in interviews. Another picture shown with pleasure was of a nephew soon to be bar-mitzvahed. Ms. B was hoping she could attend.

The usual medical problems and symptoms were reviewed, especially a foot ulcer for which she had a doctor's appointment; takes heart medicine; has diabetes; macular degeneration in right eye; some clouding of vision in left eye after a corneal transplant. Speaking of prior psychiatric hospitalizations, she seemed unphased to utter this in presence of her roommate. Asked about her appetite and eating habits, she said she "eats OK," but her roommate contradicted with "she doesn't, she eats poorly, just little bits, we cook prepared foods in the microwave." Responding to this remark that she was not a good eater, Ms. B countered that she "used to have a good appetite at one time and gained a lot of weight, now drinks 'bottled breakfasts' with milk she didn't use to like but now 'drinks a lot.'" Sleeping continues "a problem," listening to TV late into the night, rising late in the day, lying down during the day but not sleeping. "Fortunately, we are both night people."

I wondered whether she thought about mother very much. An outpouring of criticism followed of how terrible mother was to her, how she still doesn't understand it. Mother would not support her singing, even though she had a good voice; teachers suggested lessons but mother refused. If someone complimented her, mother would beat her. She said she did not cry much anymore, but roommate refuted this, offering "her mother must have been jealous of her." The story of her "second boyfriend" was recounted once again but with possible flourishes: she said that when on his way to get her, he died in a car crash from a drunken driver; mother said it was her fault for telling him to come, blaming instead of comforting her. Engaged to marry him when she was 32, she "truly loved him and had come to trust him and felt comfortable with him." On the other hand, her fiancé was "someone she didn't like but was 'pushed by mother.'" Mother was "terrible to me even though she was sweet to others, even outside the family, but especially nice to my brothers." "She always hurt me but she got upset if she hurt the boys." Again, she repeated how she was smart, was top of the class and had "lots of boyfriends" in high school.

I asked how she spent her day. Activity consisted largely of listening to radio or TV (eyesight very poor), and she enjoyed mysteries and listened to the news. Quite spontaneously, she expressed disappointment at President Clinton's impeachment and felt that the "Republicans were awful." When asked what she thought about Clinton's behavior, she said "you mean with Monica Lewinsky; she's a tramp, she pursued him, stalked him while speaking highly of him."

We talked more about her move from the nursing home she described "like a prison, glad to get out of there. There was a male nurse who was very mean." When she would see her doctor at the hospital, she "would always cry when speaking of the nursing home, how the nursing home always controlled my pills."

I typically asked whether she remembered Dr. Deutsch. She did, asked whether he were still alive and why I had asked. He first diagnosed her with anorexia many years ago, I said. She laughed and said "I think I invented it (anorexia), but now I hear about it all the time."

At the end of my visit, Ms. B once again asked about my family, my sons, and whether I had grandchildren. I did answer her before asking whether I might take a picture of her with her roommate. Laughingly, she said, "sure, I'll break the camera."

As she began to rise from the sofa, I said its softness made it difficult to stand. She said her father had a lot of good furniture but because he expected her to always live in a nursing home, he sold everything. Also, "he was devastated after mother died and wanted to get out of the home where he lived." "He used to visit me, take me to the shopping mall on occasion." But then he died of a heart attack while shaving and was found by her brother "with blood all over his face." He was 84.

I asked about her next hospital visits. She saw a social worker "on occasion when I need something." Continuing appointments were scheduled for bone density studies and other orthopedic service. Laughing, she said that one doctor calls her the "shrinking woman." In a kind of one-last-shot at mother, she attributed all her disabilities, problems and sickness to mother, even though she was "always nice to others." I once again said that I didn't think mother was always so nice, that she was a troubled woman, a disturbed mother with problems of her own. Ms. B laughed and said that she had once heard two doctors talking about her mother while Ms. B was being treated for ulcers and heard one say to the other "if I had a mother like that, I'd get ulcers too."

Both Ms. B and her roommate said I should come again soon, but it was the last time I saw them before Ms. B died three years later. Minimal medical information was obtained from medical records and her medical physician, Dr. V, who had not seen her since 2001. Dr. V found her to be a "nice person whom I liked very much." Ms. B had complained of having a succession of medical doctors but was very content with Dr. V over a period of several years.

This was my last face-to-face contact with Ms. B. For a time afterward before her death in 2002, I was able to speak with Dr. V at BIH, although her freedom to share information with me was regulated and restricted by newly established laws (HIPAA, Health Insurance Portability and Accountability Act, 1996) limiting communication about patients without their express current consent. There was, however, a rumor that Ms. B had applied for or begun visits to a day rehabilitation program and that there may have been some degree of abuse of an unknown nature by a roommate. My further attempts at learning of her living circumstances, hospital visits and ultimate death were unproductive. No public obituary appeared. Both brothers and father were deceased, negating my learning more about her from living relatives. I had recalled from conversations with her mother that Ms. B's wish was to be buried in the same cemetery next to her mother (together again!).

The prediction made by so many over the years that the patient could never be separated from mother except through death seemed fulfilled, although a kind of faux mother–daughter relationship had continued with more benignly compatible substitutes.

References

Freud, S. (1923). The ego and the id. In J. Strachey et al. (Trans.) *The Standard Edition of the Complete Psychological Works of Sigmund Freud*, vol. XIX. London: Hogarth Press, pp. 3–69.

Lipsitt, D.R. (1964). Integration clinic: an approach to the teaching and practice of medical psychology in an outpatient setting. In N.E. Zinberg (Ed.) *Psychiatry and Medical Practice in a General Hospital.* New York: International Universities Press, pp. 231–249.

Lipsitt, D.R. (1974). Psychodynamic considerations of hypochondriasis. *Psychotherapy and psychosomatics*, *23*(1–6), 132–141.

Lipsitt, D.R. (2001). Psychodynamic perspectives on hypochondriasis. In V. Starcevic & D.R. Lipsitt (Eds.) *Hypochondriasis: Modern Perspectives on an Ancient Malady*. New York: Oxford University Press, pp. 183–201.

6 The Elusive Therapeutics of Anorexia Nervosa

In the world of therapeutics, the search for workable treatments for anorexia nervosa has persisted not for decades but for centuries. As early as the 1800s, Sir William W. Gull (1874) and Ernest-Charles Lasègue (1873) identified a puzzling symptomatology of young women as most likely a psychological disorder. They encouraged support, tolerance, patience and attentive listening to family interaction as essential components of treatment, even as they experimented with lotions, hydrotherapy, medicinals and other treatments of the time. Gull advocated a holistic view of medicine and disease and offered therapeutics consisting mostly of "time and rest" even while trying cinchona, bichloride of mercury, and syrup of iodide and iron, "but no perceptible effect followed their administration" (Kaufman & Heiman, 1964, p. 133). This "tincture of time" is upheld as a part of all recommended treatments.

Anorexia nervosa had long been considered a "medical" illness, but with poor understanding of etiology and effective therapy, it increasingly became of interest to psychiatrists and psychoanalysts. It was the latter who introduced the idea of pregnancy fantasies. Probably the tendency of the disease to simulate psychoses, particularly schizophrenia, suggested to medical physicians that it was a disease beyond their competence to treat. "Indeed, approach to treatment has recently become confused owing to the mystery which now surrounds its etiology, at one time explained in terms which, if superficial, at least were easily understood" (Kaufman & Heiman, 1964, p. 191). "The discouraging results of treatment based on general medical principles is one of the more obvious causes of its [medicine's] defection" (p. 194).

A classic paper by Edward Bibring (1954) describes "therapeutic principles and procedures" of all psychotherapies, regardless of ideology. He lists suggestion, abreaction (emotional discharge), manipulation (e.g., guidance, advice, redirecting and mobilizing), clarification and interpretation. According to Bibring, the principles of suggestion, emotional discharge and manipulation do not promote "any self-understanding on the part of the patient" (p. 745). Only the techniques of clarification and

DOI: 10.4324/9781003208693-6

interpretation contribute to the development of insight and personal psychological growth, according to Bibring. These principles occur in some measure in Ms. B's experience.

Ursano, Sonnenberg, and Lazar (1991) believe that behavioral change occurs through two major therapeutic processes: understanding cognitive and affective patterns derived from childhood (defense mechanisms) and understanding the conflicted relationships one had with one's significant childhood figures as re-experienced in the doctor–patient relationship (transference). The intensity and duration of the turbulent mother–daughter relationship in Ms. B's case seemed to obstruct any appreciation of cognitive and affective patterns that would promote insight in either mother or daughter. And the fighting that occurred between them defied opportunities to explore childhood recollections that might identify strengths and weaknesses in development.

By 1984, Vandereycken and Meermann (1984, pp. 12, 13) exclaimed that "no single treatment modality, psychotherapeutic, psychopharmacology or nutritional [had] provided the final solution for the management of this intriguing syndrome" (p. 12). In their opinion,

> only by taking into account various etiology factors and their interdependence (the multidimensional view) on the one hand, and their development in the temporal course of the illness (the developmental approach) on the other, can a rational and causal therapy be effective. (p. 61)

By 2019, others had written that the cognitive behavioral approach had limited efficacy (Agras, 2019, p. 169), even with multiple therapeutic attempts and supportive management. A variety of therapies include cognitive-behavioral therapy (CBT), cognitive remediation therapy (CRT), dialectical behavioral treatment (DBT), family-based (Maudsley approach) treatment, interpersonal psychotherapy (ITP), psychodynamic psychotherapy, hospitalization (in and out), group or team treatment, and multidimensional treatment and perhaps others. In my opinion, when an abundance of therapies is advocated for a single disease, there is usually no particular "gold standard" choice, although recognition of the importance of parents has fostered a preference, by some, for family therapy.

In virtually all treatments, some percentage of patients improve, some remain the same, and some become chronic or die, usually from the ravages of starvation or intercurrent morbidity. A randomized controlled trial of three psychological treatments of anorexia (Byrne et al., 2017) showed no significant differences, although all were said to show some improvement. In 2018, Javaras and Pizzagalli (2020) noted that the "majority of patients [studied] do not meet the criteria for remission or recovery after treatment" (p. 567).

One 21-year outcome study of anorexia treatments found that 51% of patients fully recovered, 21% partially recovered, 10% still met full diagnostic criteria, and 16% deceased with a mortality rate of 9.8% (Lowe et al., 2001), percentages very nearly the same in most reported studies. Reported mortality rates vary from study to study, ranging from 5% to as much as 20%, depending on comorbidities (Kask et al., 2016).

It is this variability of treatment approaches, questionable etiologies, outcomes and cumulative statistics which makes anorexia such a challenge (Lipsitt, 1989; Savukoski, Maatta & Uusiautti, 2011). The only consistently effective approach to treatment includes urgency to achieve weight gain through acceptance of and commitment to treatment by the patient as well as the family. This must also, of course, involve an accepting, kind, empathic, non-controlling, listening therapist! Some empathic physicians may wittingly or unwittingly provide therapeutic acceptance, interest and support to potential anorexic patients without identifying the illness as such.

Satisfactory treatment of anorexia nervosa, as indicated, has long been characterized as difficult, frustrating and ineffective. A review of anorexia nervosa in 1950 (Cobb) recorded poor treatment outcomes. Beginning with the comment "The results of treatment in anorexia nervosa are poor and have not benefited from its inclusion with the psychosomatic disorders," pessimism extends throughout (Cobb, 1950, p. 193). Outcome in Cobb's (as in most other reported) series was largely unaffected by hospital treatment. Cobb's perception was that those who recovered did so of their own volition in the fullness of time, mostly after their environment had deliberately or accidentally changed. Cobb's impression was that few patients with "successfully" treated anorexia could actually state reasons for their recovery and that both circumstances of onset and recovery had a quality of whimsicality.

Cobb's article (1950) reviews treatments with and without intubation as well as the case of leucotomy, arguing against it. The study followed 53 patients, of whom 10 died, 8 from malnutrition; others recovered spontaneously; 23 recovered completely (the usual 50% noted in other studies). Starvation was the usual cause of death.

The range of recommended treatments has accumulated since that first applied centuries ago. The attentive listening and refeeding proposed by Gull and Lasègue as essential therapeutic attributes at that time characterize virtually all therapeutic approaches today. The desperate search for therapeutic interventions has included such experimental techniques as yoga and programed exercise (Landgren, 2022; Neumark-Sztainer et al., 2018).

Of this poor track record of treatment, Zhu et al. (2020) wrote: "there is an urgent need not only to strengthen our existing knowledge with studies of sufficient power; it fundamentally is also essential to derive novel conceptualizations of what 'treatment involves'" (p. 206).

My own opinion of the interviews reproduced here is that none really constituted a *bono fide* treatment other than the requisite interest, thoughtful listening, questioning and support while collecting data. Ms. B usually welcomed and responded to invitations to talk in psychological testing or psychiatric interviewing. She obviously survived all short-term encounters and lived in a chronic state to the age 83. My long-term relationship with her was one of interest, concern and support without a strong alliance or effort to cast our contacts in any theoretical model of therapy. As highlighted by Charon (2004), "the doctor with narrative skills habitually confirms the patient's worth in the process of attending seriously to what he or she tells" (p. 862). One can only speculate whether results might have differed with other "interventions."

Psychoanalytic and Psychodynamic Therapy

After Sigmund Freud's visit to America in 1909, Dr. James Jackson Putnam (1910), a Harvard neurologist (nonpsychiatrist), took great interest in the contribution that psychoanalysis could make to general medicine and psychiatry. His advocacy lent support to the psychogenic nature of anorexia nervosa, a significant advance in knowledge and clinical application in the 20th century.

Psychoanalysts for the most part have avoided this choice of treatment for anorexia. The few psychoanalytic therapy cases reported stress the challenges of transference, countertransference and inaccessibility of the patient through rejection and denial. Only rare cases appear in the literature, and eating disorder specialists like Hilde Bruch and John Sours, both trained in psychoanalysis, advise against its application. The complex transference/countertransference issues make the psychoanalytic approach daunting. Nonetheless, valuable insights have been proffered by psychoanalysts regarding developmental issues and interpersonal relations, especially with parental figures, afflicting young girls. Psychoanalytic studies shed light on attachment issues (à la Bowlby, 1969, 1978) and individuation-separation in the developmental framework essential to treatment (Birksted-Breen, 1989; Fischer, 1989).

As mentioned, even a committed psychoanalyst like Felix Deutsch (1927) cautioned that "one has to decide whether a deep-digging psychotherapeutic method like psychoanalysis should be recommended" (p. 52), although he did not decry psychoanalytically informed approaches as illustrated in his associative anamnesis technique.

The Mount Sinai Seminar Group on anorexia nervosa (Kaufman & Heiman, 1964, p. 99) did not "discard the baby with the bathwater," claiming that "psychoanalysis added to the study of adaptation a more detailed investigation of processes going on within the organism both consciously and unconsciously" (p. 99). The Group emphasized that all illness is multifactorial (e.g., genetic, trauma, regression, adaptation, sexualization, symbolism, aggression, undischarged affect, family relations, sociocultural and pathogenetic influences).

From the earliest days (Gull and Lasègue), recommendations for treatment had been rudimentary, since little else was available. Even then, "a kind but firm hand, a calm demeanor, and much patience" were considered indispensable (Charcot, 1889). Added to these "indispensable conditions" were the systematic exclusion of hydrotherapy and parents from "treatment programs." Several authors had alluded to the reassuring and supportive effects of the physician's countenance and demeanor on the patient. These fundamental attributes of treatment (except hydrotherapy) have not been ignored in current approaches to therapy with the patient with anorexia.

Because of the complicated impediments to treatment, randomized trials of therapy are rare. Problems encountered have included small samples, high drop-out rates, short-term outcomes, lack of comparability of therapies, and resistance of patients to participation. In the few studies reviewed by the Cochrane database system of 2015, "no specific treatment was consistently superior to any other specific approach" (Cochrane, 2015). However, Zipfel et al. (2014), comparing focal psychodynamic therapy with cognitive-behavioral therapy and "treatment as usual," concluded that "focal psychodynamic therapy proved advantageous" (Zipfel et al., 2014, p. 127). The Cochrane Report is not measurably different from that described by Vandereycken and Meermann in 1984 (p. 12, see above).

Rise and Fall of "Oral Impregnation" in Therapy

We do not need Freud to remind us of the formative impact of the earliest feeding experience of mother and infant. It is the point where all those with anorexia (and others) begin life. Much is yet to be plumbed about this most important phase of maturation, studied by psychoanalysts, psychologists and other researchers for many years (Winnicott, 1960; Bowlby, 1978; Lipsitt, 1977; Brazelton, 1976; Kagan, 1995; and others). Extensive literature exists on mother–child relations, while few publications focus on the relation of the infant to the breast.

Along with cardiac and pulmonary function, the earliest system function is related to the mouth, taking nourishment, expressing feelings (voice) and bonding with mother, especially while feeding at the breast. As soon as a child is born, the most immediate survival functions (besides a beating heart) are breathing and eating. Breathing is automatic but eating relies on some activity of the infant along with guidance from the mother. This involvement with survival is much more likely to become incorporated in the developing child's sense of self, affecting mental and physical growth. It is virtually impossible to know what psychological traces are left on a growing brain when a sucking infant finds no milk or when a soothing nipple is abruptly withdrawn from the infant's mouth.

Behavior, habits and symbolism related to the mouth, swallowing, chewing, biting and so on are imprinted early on the psyche and may persist for a lifetime, often unconsciously. This earliest developmental period is referred to as the "oral phase." At birth, the infant is largely a physical being who *somatizes* (i.e., expresses emotion in physical terms) all experience until, through maturation, learning and socialization, it is able to *desomatize* (use other mechanisms and functions of adjustment). Under stress, trauma or conflict, *re-somatization* is likely to occur. It is this re-somatization, referred to as regression to more infantile modes of behavior, that in extreme cases qualifies as illness (Lipsitt, 1992). These somatization processes, with many physical symptoms, permeated Ms. B's life.

As soon as the maturing child becomes aware of the presence of a pregnant mother or the birth of siblings, questions begin to be asked about the process of birth. All children develop fantasies of how babies "are made"; stories of "the stork" are soon displaced by the role of kissing, sucking, eating and the like. In the many contacts that Ms. B had with treaters, surprisingly little data emerges of early interactions of mother and infant.

With the advent of psychoanalysis and interest of psychoanalysts in patients' fantasy and symbolic language, the notion of "oral impregnation" became a topic of considerable discussion. Fear of pregnancy, in and of itself, is not pathological in most individuals except in those who are severely conflicted. Raciborski (1865) wrote that "excessive fear of pregnancy or immediate desire of bearing children...may induce more or less delay in appearance of catamenia and even a protracted state of amenorrhea" (Kaufman & Heiman, 1964, p. 25).

Much of the somatic symptomatology of anorexia centers on orality along with restricted or excessive eating, vomiting, gastrointestinal disturbances and so on. Combined with expressed wishes and fears of pregnancy or equating fatness with pregnancy, the presence of amenorrhea as a preeminent symptom of anorexia had led naturally, in analytic parlance, to a patient's expression of oral impregnation. However, review of early cases and examination of the interviews included here shows that the actual utterance of such fantasy was rare indeed, more often the *interpretation* by the treaters. Ms. B's interviews are replete with "pregnancy metaphors" but not "oral impregnation."

In the Boston Psychoanalytic Society & Institute (BPSI) seminar cited above, where Romano described his experience with the patient, Dr. Helene Deutsch related details of treatment of her own patient with anorexia. She states, "she had intense pregnancy fantasies, the picture being that of impregnation through the mouth." Deutsch adds, however, that the fantasy is less relevant than it is in hysteria "and is not an expression of an infantile theory of procreation" (see Romano's notes, BPSI seminar, December 16, 1941).

Paul Roazen's (1981) account of Dr. Helene Deutsch's remarks at this seminar is more detailed. He reproduces Dr. Deutsch's comments as follows:

> alluding to an early psychoanalytically-treated case of anorexia nervosa by New York analyst Dr. Sandor Lorand (1943) in which oral impregnation fantasies are mentioned, she states "Now the pregnancy fantasy, just as in the case presented here tonight [Romano's case], impregnation is expected through the mouth. The pregnancy fantasy is something very common in hysteria...speaking only about the eating and not about the ceremonials of eating and not eating. In a hysteric, it is a libidinous one...the fantasy is 'I want to be impregnated' usually by father, and it has the character of infantile theory which is nearly a rule in one period of development. The impregnation is through the mouth but this pregnancy has a second act...she is impregnated in identification with mother...a terrible aggression against mother that has not the character of hysteric fantasy...this is turning against the self...the impregnation becomes poisonous, destructive, therefore the food now becomes poisoned."
>
> (Roazen, 1981, p. 506)

Deutsch focuses more on the importance of obsessionalism and ceremonials and thinks she suggested "pregnancy" to her patient, causing her to report when she buys a new dress that she looks pregnant. Deutsch states: "It was an acting out of what she has learned in analysis, but it has not any therapeutic influence," mirroring remarks by Bruch about psychoanalytic treatment.

Fantasies of oral impregnation are again referred to in the paper by Waller, Kaufman and Deutsch (1940). They state that "the symbolism of eating as impregnation is quite clear and unambiguous" (Kaufman & Heiman, 1964, p. 271). Although Kaufman was a co-author of this paper, his postscript candidly evaluates the emphasis on oral impregnation, suggesting that its therapeutic value has perhaps been overdetermined and that it is only one factor in a speculative psychodynamic formulation in cases of anorexia where symptoms of constipation and amenorrhea contribute to echoes of pregnancy. The overdetermination, he says, is intended only to "stress the significance of symbolizations in physiological functions" (Kaufman & Heiman, 1964, p. 246). He writes that

> The authors... attempt[ed] to utilize analytic concepts especially in relation to the content of the fantasy, and to give meaning to the signs and symptoms of the syndrome, relating it to content and utilizing the generally accepted psychoanalytic hypotheses...The patient's remarks pointing to ideas of oral impregnation were *merely indications or clues* (my emphasis) of underlying ideation.
>
> (p. 247)

Since "very little material concerning the early life in terms of preconscious or unconscious fantasy is known, it becomes necessary to *extrapolate constructions* (my emphasis) from chronologically later experiences to the early phase of development" (p. 247). Kaufman repeatedly "stresses the hypothetical nature of the oral impregnation fantasy and that the absence of data...forces a speculation rather than a deduction based on convincing clinical data" (p. 249).

In 1942, Dr. Ruth Moulton, a prominent New York psychoanalyst, reported her therapeutic experience with four cases of anorexia in *Psychosomatic Medicine* (Moulton, 1942). She heavily relied on the idea of oral impregnation fantasies as *basic* to the anorexia syndrome. She attributes rejection of food intake to fears of pregnancy. Menses are suppressed in relation to the fantasy and "the child in the abdomen is expressed through constipation" (Kaufman & Heiman, 1964, p. 276). The symptom of vomiting is described by Moulton as the wish to reject pregnancy through the gastrointestinal tract. In a summarizing comment, Moulton states "anorexia nervosa is...a psychosomatic entity in which fantasies of oral impregnation are dramatized through starvation, vomiting, and amenorrhea" (Kaufman & Heiman, 1964, p. 295).

Since no report of actual interviews is included in Moulton's paper, it is difficult to know whether patients actually described oral impregnation fantasies or they are rather inferred, as implied by Kaufman, through the analyst's interpretations of interview material. She states that the "common purposes of starvation are to prevent the onset of menses, prevent pregnancy, and prevent growing up" (p. 293). Interestingly, she concludes that "therapy in anorexia nervosa is most unsatisfactory" (p. 295). She states that "long hospitalization in adolescence [at least a year] is recommended because of extreme resistance and neurotic parental attitudes" (Kaufman & Heiman, 1964, p. 297).

In the 1950 article on anorexia nervosa by Cobb, much discussion ensues among participants caring for cases of anorexia. Of 16 cases reported in this paper, only one expressed ideas of oral impregnation. The likelihood is noted that such fantasies exist in all children but are probably repressed very soon. The mouth as a source of sexual and erotic significance is certainly not dismissed. Cobb wondered whether "the suggestion of this idea [fantasy of oral impregnation] by a psychiatrist could be completely ruled out" (Cobb, 1950, p. 166). On the other hand, Dr. Lucie Jessner (to whom Ms. B had been referred by Waller) suggested that "how eating means impregnation will be the mainstay of therapy," "working through with the patient these fantasies" (Cobb, 1950, p. 169). Cobb concludes, "certainly fear of pregnancy is common enough and in conflict with the normal and powerful desire to have a baby. Such fantasies and conflicts may well be important in the psychological background of anorexia nervosa" (p. 180).

The reader will observe in the content of interviews replicated here that there is hardly a mention of oral pregnancy by the patient. Furthermore, discussion of treatment later suggests that oral impregnation is rarely alluded to and that, in fact, the relevance of such symbolization or fantasy is now rarely advised as a component of treatment. In a 1975 interview (Roche Report, April 19 1975), Bruch, trained in psychoanalysis, is quoted: "[interpretations] have worked to death the concept of orality and fear of oral impregnation" (p. 8). John Rickman, a British psychoanalyst, while not specifically speaking of the fantasy of oral impregnation, comments that

> the impact of the phantasy (sic) life of one person on another is always strong—the creations of the artist, the power of the lover, the deeds of the criminal, and the symptoms of the neurotic—hold the imagination through the fantasies thus aroused. In meeting the neurotic on his own ground of passions unfulfilled, of anxieties and of guilt, the physician shoulders a heavy task.
>
> (Rickman, 1939, p. 67)

A classic publication by Robert Lindner (1955), *The Fifty Minute Hour*, describes how the powerful influence that a patient has on his analyst can "seduce" him to join in his patient's delusional fantasies.

As new research paths pursue endocrinologic, physiologic and neurological answers to the illness and behavior patterns of the patient with anorexia, the notion of "oral impregnation" has virtually disappeared from the literature.

Pharmacological Treatment

As mentioned, both Gull and Lasègue advocated "time and rest" rather than medicinals, although "tonics" and "nourishing diet" were used with paced refeedings. Medicinals of the times (Kaufman & Heiman, 1964, p. 133) were all to no avail. Gull wrote that with "warmth and steady supplies of food and stimulants, the strength may be gradually resuscitated, and recovery completed" (p. 135), recovery occurring within 2 years' time. Gull said "nursing and food," not drugs, were most important.

Since Gull's failed efforts, use of drugs as a therapeutic intervention has been advised against except in instances where anxiety or depression is an accompanying major symptom, and there is some alleged benefit from olanzapine (Dunican & DelDotto, 2007) and others, but most writers acknowledge their ineffectiveness. Even Morton was alleged to have tried "aromatic bags," "bitter medicines" and "antihysterick waters" on his early patients (Minuchin et al., 1978, p. 12).

In spite of Gull's caution, searches for pharmacological remedies persist, usually with little or no success. Controlled studies of pharmacological treatments of anorexia have been sparse. A study of dronabinol (synthetic cannabinoid agonist) administered over a 4-week period in severe enduring anorexia nervosa "induced a small but significant grain (sic) in the absence of severe adverse events" (Andries et al., 2014).

I had also been enticed to try the pharmacological agent prolixin with perhaps no more than placebo benefit (for both patient and myself!). I must have considered Ms. B's symptomatology and behavior a kind of faux-psychosis, the indication for use of such a drug. The drug was soon discontinued as noncontributory to treatment.

Ascendance of Family Therapy

Clinical experience with patients with anorexia cites family interactions fostering and/or sustaining the illness (Yager, 1982). Because of the salient role of the mother in anorexic illness, therapists began including families in treatment. Minuchin was an early investigator of the role of family therapy in treatment of anorexia nervosa. Minuchin began constructing a family therapy model in the 1960s that became best known in the 1970s with the co-authored book *Psychosomatic Families* (Minuchin et al., 1978).

Studies appeared with greater frequency in both professional and public media. An article in the *Archives of General Psychiatry* (Lock et al., 2010) states that the families of adolescent patients with anorexia nervosa were being included more and more often in the treatment of the disorder. The study found that having cooperative parents supervise each meal to make sure their child eats may be more efficacious than traditional one-on-one treatment with a therapist. As an early proponent of a psychodynamic form of family therapy in what he called "psychosomatic families," Minuchin stated, "the anorectic's behavior is determined by the degree and type of controlled interaction between the anorectic (patient) and her parents" (Sours, 1980, p. 321).

The evolution of family therapy (the Maudsley approach, named after the London hospital where it was developed) was advocated by Minuchin as a desired treatment. Application of family therapy attracted "breakthrough" media attention when *U.S. News & World Report* (Sohn, 2002) featured a story on "*Anorexia in the Family*." Some therapists considered the treatment the "gold standard" for anorexia therapy. The study of patients with anorexia (Lock et al., 2010) found that "121 patients with anorexia were randomly assigned to one of two treatments." "At six months, 40 percent in family-based treatment were in full remission versus 18 percent in individual therapy. At one year, the numbers were 49 percent and 23 percent, respectively" (p. 1029). The family therapy explored in this study focused on parents actively helping kids learn to eat and gain weight, then turning more autonomy over to the patients as their functioning improves.

Sir Arthur Crisp, a British researcher in anorexia nervosa, suggested that family-based treatment may benefit teens with anorexia. Crisp nonetheless cautioned that "outlook is poor, for about half remain chronically ill and the average length of illness in those who eventually recover is about 4 years. Almost 1 in 20 people with such severe anorexia nervosa will die from it" (Crisp, 1983, p. 856). Although outcome is not good, the best treatment according to Crisp is that which at least keeps patients alive.

More than 35 years later, *Psychiatric News* (Walsh, 2021) stated, "there have been no dramatic developments in our knowledge of how to treat individuals with eating disorders." Walsh ranks "family-based treatment (Maudsley method) [as] most promising in the last quarter century." Echoing Crisp's realistic assessment, Walsh states that even with family therapy involving parent-focused treatment, "relapse is substantial."

With Ms. B as described here, many physicians (both psychiatric and nonpsychiatric) had predicted that the patient could not get well unless she and mother could be therapeutically involved or "until the mother died." In fact, her longevity (and chronicity) may largely be due to the mother's death in the late 1960s of lymphoma at age 69. All psychiatrists and social workers familiar with mother asserted that neither mother nor daughter was a likely candidate for family approaches because of serious psychopathology between them.

Supportive Treatment

Virtually all interventions that help patients maintain control and avoid comorbidities, starvation and the like might be called supportive in nature, contributing, as Arthur Crisp has said, to keeping the patient alive. It is likely that most of the "interventions" that Ms. B received in her long course might be characterized thus. Perhaps social interaction is underappreciated as an essential attribute of "total treatment." Whether teachers, nurses, doctors, nursing home staff and acquaintances and a pet cat may all have contributed to keeping the patient alive is a moot point. Conversely, isolation is known to have adverse effects on illness and survival (Harari, 2014).

The sadomasochistic, mutually dependent relationship with mother that dominated her entire illness might be considered the "social" aspect of Ms. B's experience but, in some mystical way, may have sustained her. A kind of marginal adaptation, much below her early promise, seems achieved, as many predicted, only with mother's death. The salient and potentially beneficial feature of Ms. B's contacts with any of her treaters may be attributed to interest, respect, concern and support, in no small measure basic aspects of a "therapeutic" experience. My interactions with Ms. B over many years were sporadic and intermittent yet sufficient to prompt mother to allow that "he is the best psychiatrist she has had."

I would make occasional interpretations about how she reacted to me or to nursing home helpers as she would to mother, with only a flickering spark of insight, appearing to have little therapeutic impact. Experientially, she lived out her life by eventually finding a woman companion with whom she lived in low-cost housing in a "mother-like" but much less destructive relationship.

Acknowledging the difficulties in achieving progress in this most difficult group of patients, virtually all researchers urge better studies, larger pools of subjects, longer treatment and outcome results, difficult as these objectives are with this population of patients with anorexia.

References

Agras, W.S. (2019). Cognitive behavior therapy for the eating disorders. *Psychiatric Clinics of North America*, 42(2), 169–179.

Andries, A., Frystyk, J., Flyvbjerg, A., & Steving, R.K. (2014). Dronabinol in severe, enduring anorexia nervosa: a randomized controlled trial. *International Journal of Eating Disorders*, 47(1), 18–23.

Bibring, E. (1954). Psychoanalysis and the dynamic psychotherapies. *Journal of the American Psychoanalytic Association*, 2, 745–770.

Birksted-Breen, D. (1989). Working with an anorexic patient. *American Journal of Psychoanalysis*, 70(Pt 1), 29–39.

Bowlby, J. (1969). *Attachment and Loss I: Attachment*. New York: Basic Books.

Bowlby, J. (1978). Attachment theory and its therapeutic implications. *Adolescent Psychiatry*, 6, 5–33.

Brazelton, T.B. (1976). The parent-infant attachment. *Clinical Obstetrics and Gynecology*, 19(2), 373–389.

Bruch, H. (1975). How to treat anorexia nervosa. *Roche Report. Frontiers of Psychiatry*, April 15, 5(8), 1–11, p. 2.

Byrne, S., Wade, T., Hay, P., Touyz, S., Fairburn, C.G., Treasure, J., Schmidt, U., McIntosh, V., Allen, K., Fursland, A., & Crosby, R.D. (2017). A randomised controlled trial of three psychological treatments for anorexia nervosa. *Psychological Medicine*, 47(16), 2823–2833.

Charcot, J.M. (1889). *Diseases of the Nervous System*. London: The New Sydenham Society, pp. 210–211.

Charon, R. (2004). Narrative and medicine. *New England Journal of Medicine*, 350(9), 862–864.

Cobb, S., & Reid, J.R. (1950). *Emotions and Clinical Medicine*. New York: W.W. Norton and Co.

Cochrane Database System Review 2015(7) CD 003909, P. Hay et al).

Crisp, A.H. (1983). Regular review: anorexia nervosa. *British Medical Journal*, 287, 855–858.

Deutsch, F. (1927). Psychoanalysis and internal medicine. In M.R. Kaufman & M. Heiman (Eds.) (1964) *Evolution of Psychosomatic Concepts: Anorexia Nervosa: A Paradigm*. New York: International Universities Press, Inc., pp. 47–55.

Dunican, K.C., & DelDotto, D. (2007). The role of olanzapine in the treatment of anorexia nervosa. *Annals of Pharmacotherapy*, 41(1), 111–115.

Fischer, N. (1989). Anorexia nervosa and unresolved rapprochement conflicts: a case study. *International Journal of Psychoanalysis*, 70(Pt i), 41–54.

Gull, W.W. (1874). Anorexia nervosa (apepsia hysterica, anorexia hysterica). *Transactions of the Clinical Society of London*, 7, 221–228.

Harari, E. (2014) Supportive psychotherapy. *Australasia Psychiatry*, 22(5), 440–442.

Javaras, K.N., & Pizzagalli, D.A. (2020). Neural insensitivity to the effects of hunger: a potential mechanism underlying persistent dietary restriction in anorexia nervosa? *American Journal of Psychiatry*, 177(7), 567–569.

Kagan, J. (1995). On attachment. *Harvard Review of Psychiatry*, 3(2), 104–106.

Kask, J., Ekselius, L., Brandt, L., Kollia, N., Ekbom, A., & Pepadopoulus, F.C. (2016). Mortality in women with anorexia nervosa: the role of comorbid psychiatric disorders. *Psychosomatic Medicine*, 78(8), 910–919.

Kaufman, M.R., & Heiman, M. (1964). *Evolution of Psychosomatic Concepts: Anorexia Nervosa: A Paradigm*. New York: International Universities Press, Inc., p. 25

Landgren, K. (2022). Ear acupuncture as an adjunct in a treatment protocol for anorexia nervosa: utilization rate and nurses' experience. *Acupuncture Medicine*, 40(4), 322–332.

Lasègue, C. (1873). On hysterical anorexia (*De l'Anorexie Hysterique*). *Medical Times and Gazette*, 2, 265–266, 367–369.

Lindner, R. (1955). *The Fifty-Minute Hour: A Collection of True Psychoanalytic Tales*. New York: Generic.

Lipsitt, D.R. (1989). Anorexia nervosa, Felix Deutsch, and the associative anamnesis: a psychosomatic kaleidoscope. *Psychosomatic Medicine*, 51, 597–601.

Lipsitt, D.R. (1992). Challenges of somatization: diagnostic, therapeutic and economic. *Psychiatry in Medicine*, 10(3), 1–12.

Lipsitt, L.P. (1977). The study of sensory and learning processes of the newborn. *Clinical Periinatology*, 4(1), 163–186.

Lock, J., Le Grange, D., Agras, S., Moye, A., Bryson, S.W., & Jo, B. (2010). Randomized clinical trial comparing family-based treatment of adolescent-focused individual therapy for adolescents with anorexia nervosa. *Archives of General Psychiatry*, 67(10), 1025–1032.

Lorand, S. (1943). Anorexia nervosa: report of a case. *Psychosomatic Medicine*, 5, 282–292.

Lowe, B., Zipfel, S., Buchholz, C., Dupont, Y., Reas, D.L., & Herzog, W. (2001). Long-term outcome of anorexia nervosa in a prospective 21-year follow-up study. *Psychological Medicine*, 31(5), 881–890.

Minuchin, S., Rosman, B.L., & Baker, L. (1978). *Psychosomatic Families: Anorexia Nervosa in Context*. Cambridge, MA: Harvard University Press.

Moulton, R. (1942). A psychosomatic study of anorexia nervosa including the use of vaginal smears. *Psychosomatic Medicine*, 4, 62–74. Also in M.R. Kaufman & M. Heiman (Eds.) (1964) *Evolution of Psychosomatic Concepts: Anorexia Nervosa: A Paradigm*. New York: International Universities Press, Inc., pp. 274–297.

Neumark-Sztainer, D., Watts, A.W., & Rydell, S. (2018). Yoga and body image: how do young adults practicing yoga describe its impact on their body image? *Body Image*, 27, 156–168.

Putnam, J.J. (1910). Personal impressions of Sigmund Freud: his work and special reference to his recent lectures at Clarke University. *Journal of Abnormal Psychology*, 46(6), 372–379.

Raciborski, A. (1865). *De l'amenorr par causes psychiques. Archives de Medicinehee*, 1, 529. In M.R. Kaufman & M. Heiman (Eds.) (1964) *Evolution of Psychosomatic Concepts: Anorexia Nervosa: A Paradigm*. New York: International Universities Press, Inc., p. 25.

Rickman, J. (1939). The general practitioner and psychoanalysis. In W. Clifford & M. Scott (Ed.) (1957) *Selected Contributions to Psychoanalysis*. London: The Hogarth Press, pp. 61–67.

Roazen, P. (1981). Anorexia nervosa: Helene Deutsch, M.D. *Bulletin of the Menninger Clinic*, 45(6), 499–501.

Savukoski, M, Maatta, K., & Uusiautti, S. (2011). The other side of well-being—what makes a young woman become an anorectic? *International Journal of Psychological Studies*, 3(2), 76–87.

Sohn, E. (2002). Anorexia in the family. *U.S. News and World Report*, June 10.

Sours, J.A. (1980). *Starving to Death in a Sea of Objects: The Anorexia Nervosa Syndrome*. New York: Jason Aronson.

Ursano, R.J., Sonnenberg, S.M., & Lazar, S.G. (1991). *Concise Guide to Psychodynamic Psychotherapy*. Arlington, VA: American Psychiatric Publishing Inc.

Vandereycken, W., & Meermann, R. (1984). *Anorexia Nervosa: A Clinician's Guide to Treatment*. Berlin, Germany: De Gruyter.

Waller, J.V., Kaufman, M.R., & Deutsch, F. (1940). Anorexia nervosa: a psychosomatic entity. *Psychosomatic Medicine*, 2, 3–16.

Walsh, B.T. (2021). Eating disorders: current knowledge and treatment update. *Psychiatric News*, February 2021, 56(2), 19.

Winnicott, D.W. (1960). The theory of the parent-child relationship. *International Journal of Psychoanalysis*, 41, 585–595.

Yager, J. (1982). Family issues in the pathogenesis of anorexia nervosa. *Psychosomatic Medicine*, 44(1), 43–60.

Zhu, J., Yang, Y., Touyz, S., Park, R., & Hay, P. (2020). Psychological treatments for people with severe and enduring anorexia nervosa: a mini review. *Frontiers in Psychiatry*, 11, 206, 1–8.

Zipfel, S., Wild, B., Grosz, G., Friedrich, H.C., et al. (2014). Focal psychodynamic therapy, cognitive behavior therapy, and optimized treatment as usual in outpatients with anorexia nervosa (ANTOP study): randomized controlled trial. *Lancet*, 383(9912), 127–137.

7 Summing Up

> What is a normal child like? Does he just eat and grow and smile sweetly? No, that is not what he is like. The normal child, if he has confidence in mother and father, pulls out all the stops. In the course of time, he tries out his power to disrupt, to destroy, to frighten, to wear down, to waste, to wangle, and to appropriate...At the start he absolutely needs to live in a circle of love and strength (with consequent tolerance) if he is not to be too fearful of his own thoughts and of his imaginings to make progress in his emotional development.
>
> –D.W. Winnicott, 1992, p. 124

"Flashback": A Retrospective Glance

August 22, 2019. On this anniversary date, Ms. B would have been 100 years old. Her story spans nearly my entire career. Her mother haunts me, as she haunted her daughter. In the long, contentious relationship between mother and daughter, it is virtually impossible to know which "child" (à la Winnicott, see above) mother was responding to.

My acquaintance with Ms. B has been an education. It has burnished my interest in psychosomatic medicine and complex and difficult-to-treat cases. Her illness has drawn me to anorexia nervosa but has not made me an expert in that field. I had no illusions about "rescuing" this one patient, only that I was captivated by this puzzling disease and I liked her. Through her, I became acquainted with some of the luminaries in American psychiatry. (Dr. Felix Deutsch had corresponded with me and expressed interest in my account but unfortunately died early [1964] as the story was evolving.) See Figures A3.1 and A3.2 for correspondence with Dr. Felix Deutsch about Ms. B.

With a story that covers 64 years, during 41 of which I had personally known her, what have I learned? While much can be gleaned from the copious literature on anorexia nervosa, Ms. B provides an encyclopedia of knowledge about her own life experience and her struggles with a difficult mother. During my first residency year, my chief, Dr. Milton Rosenbaum, dissuaded trainees from spending too much time with books

DOI: 10.4324/9781003208693-7

since "you can learn almost everything you have to know about psychiatry by working with one patient for a year."

As physicians, we do not need to cure every ill to have an impact on patients' lives. It is no revelation that not all therapeutic efforts are effective. Giving up in the face of frustration, resistance, disappointment or anger is not part of the physician's armamentarium, although some practitioners have questioned how persevering one must be in refractory cases (Hawkins, 2021; Sawhill et al., 2020; Schneiderman et al., 1990).

In an illness with notoriously high mortality rates, biological and physiological threats to survival are abundant; threats of suicide and homicide in this case greatly increased that risk. The fact that Ms. B had lived to 83 may be testimony to her own resilience but also to the "assist" provided over time by her various "caretakers," including internists, surgeons, endocrinologists, orthopedists, psychiatrists, social workers, psychologists and nurses, a panoply of practitioners which represents considerable resource consumption. One may question how well she might have done without all such assistance.

Comparing Ms. B's story with that described in the literature on anorexia nervosa, we can say that she was in no way typical. There was no evidence of the "relentless pursuit of thinness," nor was there a pronounced preoccupation with body image, except when she was concerned about how she might look to others. A kind of marginal adaptation, much below her early promise, seems achieved only with mother's death! The salient and potentially beneficial features of Ms. B's contacts with any of her treaters can be attributed to interest, respect, concern and support, in no small way aspects of a "therapeutic" experience. My interactions with her over many years were sporadic. Although I would make occasional interpretations about how she reacted to me or to helpers in the nursing home as she would to mother, these "interpretive" comments seemed to have little impact, only occasionally a suggestive spark of insight.

No clinical and theoretical psychologist would dispute the profound significance of the first three years of life in a person's development. Some child psychologists say the very first year of an infant's life with the birth mother is most highly determinative of what will ensue in subsequent years (Brazelton, 1976; Kagan, 1995; Lipsitt, 1977; Raju, 2011).

Whether one subscribes to Sigmund Freud's theory of psychosexual development with a focus on orality, Erik Erikson's eight stages of human development with early trust or distrust, John Bowlby's theories of attachment and separation, Gordon Allport's theory of trait development, Michael Balint's theory of basic trust or any other model, all support the premise that the earliest experience of intimacy between mother and infant will be the basis for future enhancement of a mature being. When developmental deficiencies of body or mind arise, motivated individuals may take themselves to an appropriate therapist, whose task – physical, social or psychological – is to help correct developmental misadventures through assistance in adapting, revising, understanding, rejecting or accepting. Access to therapists who can meld both mind (psyche) and body (soma) in psychosomatic care is sometimes rare indeed (Winnicott, 1966).

In the case of Ms. B, we know that she was born to an immigrant mother of no prior birthing experience (other than her own) before giving birth to her first child, a daughter. Little of their very first interaction is known except through cumulative retrospective assumptions. We know that little Ms. B was born into a household of limited means, of parents with a "loveless marriage," from a mother with her own repository of mental and physical concerns. Interviews suggest that the child began life as a happy, intelligent and accomplished child, with much promise noted by teachers and others outside the home. In our most charitable accepting attitude, we can assume that the mother did have her child's welfare at heart, that she wanted to give to her, to be encouraging and loving. But all evidence in subsequent encounters suggests that she was experienced by her daughter as a very disturbed, narcissistic, hostile, angry, competitive and jealous mother, whose almost every gesture perverted any loving relationship. She deprived her daughter of the impetus of progressing to further stages of development, especially that of autonomy, self-control, initiative and industry; any efforts in that direction were usually thwarted by a conflicted and contemptuous mother. A profile of mother's behavior reflects citations in the literature of the pivotal role of a mother's interaction with her child. Summarizing the writings on mother–child relationships, Goshen-Gottstein (1986) collates the writings of Brody, Winnicott, Robertson, Blank, Stern, Pringle, Klaus and Kennell with the statement:

> A mother has to be attentive to the child's needs (food, sleep, warmth, movement, comfort, company, love, protection, control, stimulation), must not misunderstand or confuse them (to have empathy with him or her) and must fulfill them by adapting her actions to those of the child.
> (p. 55)

Furthermore,

> a key dimension of mother's behavior ('sensitivity to the infant's signals') during the baby's first year of life…to help the infant get pleasure from his or her strivings and eventually to master them…thus, in the very early stages, the mother is responsible for preparing a setting in which maturational processes are unimpeded as little as possible and object relations can develop.
> (p. 55)

It is abundantly transparent that Mrs. B did not provide such a growth-promoting environment for her daughter. The daughter, held tightly to a mutually interdependent relationship, was never able to break the deleterious bond except through the potential of death (natural, suicide or homicide), a separation ultimately replaced with "surrogate" mothers of a similar (if more benign) stripe. She managed a brief "loveless marriage," echoing mother's own life. Whatever resilience Ms. B possessed must have permitted her to live an unusually long, marginal life after an initial diagnosis of anorexia nervosa, marking her as one surviving with the chronicity of a perilously mortal disease. Were her "therapeutic encounters" helpful in that regard, or did she retain enough of her original "givens" to sustain herself through lifelong developmental insults? Perhaps a late-life renewed relationship with father and brothers after mother's death and the fact that she was liked by others such as nurses and doctors ultimately helped solve previously "unresolvable" conflicts. Questions of this kind most likely are not easily answerable.

If we could transport ourselves to before Ms. B was seen by Dr. Deutsch and Dr. Waller, we might have observed an early tumultuous family scene predictive of the trajectory of the next 64 years. Although both parent and child declared that the earliest years were "normal," the intricacies of family interaction cannot be measurably assessed. But the patient was the first-born to a mother with medical problems who wanted a baby only because her "sister had one." Father was injured in the army during World War I and may have suffered an undiagnosed case of post-traumatic stress disorder. Both parents were from Europe and may have been affected by Nazi atrocities of the times, never mentioned in interviews with patient or mother. How can one define the vectors that touched off the "spark" of anorexia nervosa? Weight loss extremes seemed associated more with social conditions and desire for control, especially with mother and dating, than with "relentless pursuit of thinness." "Rewards" of starvation from "dating and dieting" coincided with mother's reactive behavior. We have data mostly following the diagnosis of anorexia nervosa but very little before.

Interaction of parents and patient, reconstructed from social workers' notes, begins with "referral for camp placement." Ms. B was sent to camp, where she soon complained of being lonely and cried a lot. Mother promptly withdrew her, claiming that other girls criticized her daughter for always being too slow. Once home, Ms. B regretted leaving camp, asked to return for two weeks at the end of August. This request disturbed mother, who cried and seemed agitated, eliciting the comment that she was tormented by Ms. B's presence at home and did not appreciate what had been done for her at camp, criticizing her for having left. They irritated each other, she said. In August, Ms. B was not accepted back at camp "because the director felt she was a bad influence on other girls." At that point, the "case was closed" (but later reopened) since "everything had been tried and there was nothing else to do."

The patient was a young, attractive, thin, well-dressed, apprehensive girl. She had graduated high school with honors and was very popular. She held several short-term jobs. According to mother, Ms. B always had been "given her own way," and mother believed she herself was very good to her. Habitually, the girl slept from 4 a.m. to 3 p.m. When she had a date, she would come home, put her clothes away, brush her coat, clean the kitchen and maybe eat something although she didn't like to eat at home. She seemed at times anxious to be helped and willing to leave home, but these motives were always evanescent and undermined, according to a social worker.

A 40-year-old Russian-born woman with an accent was readily able to express herself in English. She seemed extremely apprehensive about her daughter, constantly attending to and dominating her. Mother was not cooperative with suggestions and insisted she could accomplish more at home by persistently keeping after her. She said she was willing to "make every sacrifice" to help her daughter return to normal. According to one social worker, "Mrs. B has a great need to have her daughter at home and also Ms. B has great difficulty detaching herself from mother."

Arrangements were made to have the girl go for medical review to an intermediary hospital where she "improved in a routinized setting." However, mother withdrew her because the place was "not clean enough for her daughter" and "she would not get sufficient attention there." She was told by the social worker that the hope was to have Ms. B "experience doing for herself."

When Ms. B visited the Endocrine Clinic several months later, the case was again reopened.

What of the Future for Anorexia Nervosa?

Many questions arise. How far have we come in understanding and combating this mystifying risky disease? (Bulik et al., 2007; Zipfel et al., 2015). Has its prevalence changed? What are today's mortality data? What more is known of its etiology than was known in the days of Sir William W. Gull and Ernest-Charles Lasègue? (Steinhausen, 2002). Indeed, in 1950, Cobb and Reid marveled that "the wonder is that Gull's purely clinical description has stood the test of time for so long" (Cobb and Reid, 1950, p. 175). With so few long-term outcome studies (Lowe et al., 2001), there is hope in the findings of a Swedish study (Dobrescu et al., 2020) in a 30-year follow-up wherein there were no deaths in the 51 patients studied, although one in five developed chronic disease.

With all our new technology and medical knowledge, are treatment outcomes improving? The disease entity called anorexia nervosa was slow to be recognized as a crisis until the 1960s (Frazier, 1963; Vandereycken & Lowenkopf, 1990), and there is concern that the crisis persists (Kaye & Bulik, 2021). Few clinicians were known for their interest and therapeutic efforts to address the perplexing illness. Hilde Bruch, Phillipa Hay, Arthur Crisp, Shervert Frazier, Katherine Halmi, John Nemiah and Stanley Cobb are a few early writers on the subject.

The fact that the illness is characterized by a multitude of both psychological and medical/endocrinologic symptoms has allowed the research and treatment pendulum to swing between medical and psychiatric hospitalizations and treatments. Because the diagnosis was so often missed by the general practitioner or family physician, the disease seemed to fall more prominently in the psychiatric domain.

With the cornucopia of available treatments, proven efficacy of one over another continues to be debated (Hay, 2020), although anecdotal accounts espouse superiority of individual therapists' preferred approaches (Bulik et al., 2007). Depending on selected studies, mortality and survival rates remain rather constant. Randomized studies in this illness are scant, given the difficulties of recruiting, sustaining, measuring and matching patients and controls (Hay et al., 2003). A systematic review of all studies in all languages from 1980 to 2005 (Bulik et al., 2007) discouragingly reported that "evidence for anorexia nervosa treatment is weak" whether medication only, behavioral interventions only or combination treatments. According to the authors, "literature [on successful treatments] is sparse and inconclusive." Only family therapy showed some efficacious results. A 2015 controlled study of inpatient treatment (Madden et al., 2015) found no benefit of length of hospitalization compared with standard medical stabilization and weight restoration in young patients with anorexia. Shorter hospitalization combined with manualized family-based treatment was recommended. All researchers, regardless of findings and because of the high mortality rate in eating disorders, encourage "future robust studies [to] inform physicians of the predictive factors associated with mortality rates in patients with eating disorders NOS (not otherwise specified) and bulimia with anorexia having the only clear predictive value of death among these disorders" (Arcelus et al., 2011; Brauser, 2011).

Ms. B of this report showed many of the prognostic indices of anorexia nervosa. There is no evidence of a "relentless pursuit of thinness," no grave concern about imminent mortality except for reciprocal threats of homicide and suicide by both mother and daughter, unlikely qualifications for successful individual or family-based therapy. What light can this case shed on insights for future directions? What is learned from this long outcome report?

Promise of Future Success?

Even Freud, the master of the "talking cure," predicted that one day the answers to mental illness would derive from chemistry, endocrinology and physiology. These fields, in addition to the continuing pursuit of more effective treatments, appear to be prominent vistas of future research into etiology and course of anorexia nervosa. Impressive advances in psychosomatic medicine and other fields of medicine in recent decades have attracted researchers to pursue answers to these unflagging questions.

This is not the place to review extensive research into possible causes of anorexia nervosa, only to welcome the urgent search for answers to a disease with high mortality and serious consequences for family and patient. Such explorations are tedious, difficult and expensive and do not readily reveal findings applicable to quotidian clinical challenge. As noted by Thomas Insel (2022a), former head of the U.S. National Institute of Mental Health, "the country's long spell without breakthrough treatments and outcomes for life's more serious diseases can be attributed, in part, to the complexity of the brain." Insel (2022b), however, does not dismiss the possibility that progress can still be made in fields like psychopharmacology for treatment of depression, schizophrenia and psychosis. To date, however, psychopharmacology has not been a pathway to successful outcomes for anorexia nervosa.

ENVOI

Early papers attributed the etiology of anorexia nervosa to unfavorable environmental influences (see chlorosis) prior to puberty as well as traumatic emotional states/experiences. While those vectors remain prominent, other etiologies are sought for this symptom complex since therapeutic attention to the former has not yielded good outcomes. Increased awareness of the impact of family dynamics has shifted therapeutic attention to involvement of families.

Ever since Bowlby (1978) proposed an attachment theory and its relevance to disease, its contribution to understanding the mother–daughter relationship in the origins of anorexia nervosa has been paramount.

One cannot fathom all the possible interactions between Mrs. B and her daughter from pre-term, birth and immediate postpartum. However, from what we do know, we can surmise a troubled and tangled reverberating circuit between an inexperienced (and conflicted) first-time mother with a new first child. Opportunities for secure and comforting early attachment were not abundantly forthcoming. Whether there were other extenuating circumstances (e.g., impoverishment and social anxiety related to war) can only be conjectured. The child was born into a poor immigrant family impacted by time of war, a father injured in the army, a societal depression and uncertainties of existence in a war-weary world.

Whatever the concatenation of events, circumstances did not bode well for secure attachment of a helpless newborn to a mother in a "loveless marriage." The interviews presented here provide ample evidence of an embattled relationship of both mother and child in endless revelatory (at times convoluted, confused, and conflictual) remarks (Winnicott, 1960).

References

Arcelus, J., Mitchell, A.J., Wales, J., & Nielsen, S. (2011). Mortality rates in patients with anorexia nervosa and other eating disorders. A meta-analysis of 36 studies. *Archives of General Psychiatry*, 68(7), 724–731.

Bowlby, J. (1978). Attachment theory and its therapeutic implications. *Adolescent Psychiatry*, 6, 5–33.

Brauser, D. (2011). All eating disorders can be deadly, anorexia the worst. *Medscape Medical News*, July 27.

Brazelton, T.B. (1976). The parent-infant attachment. *Clinical Obstetrics and Gynecology*, 19(2), 373–389.

Bulik, C.M., Berkman, N.D., Brownley, K.A., Sedway, J.A., & Lohr, K.N. (2007). Anorexia nervosa treatment: a systematic review of randomized controlled trials. *International Journal of Eating Disorders*, 40(4), 310–320.

Cobb, S., & Reid, J.R. (1950). *Emotions and Clinical Medicine*. New York: W.W. Norton and Co.

Dobrescu, S.R., Dinkler, S., Gillberg, C., Rastam, M., Gillberg, C., & Wentz, E. (2020). Anorexia nervosa: 30-year outcome. *British Journal of Psychiatry*, 216, 97–104.

Frazier, S.H. (1963). Everything on anorexia. "Anorexia nervosa held to be medical crisis." *Medical Tribune*, p. 5.

Goshen-Gottstein, E.R. (1986). On whose needs does mother focus? Mother- or child-centered care and the self-differentiation of maternal needs. *Psychiatry*, 49, 54–68.

Hawkins, J. (2021). Why even a liberal can justify limited paternalistic intervention in anorexia nervosa. *Philosophy, Psychiatry & Psychology*, 28(2), 155–158.

Hay, P. (2020). Current approach to eating disorders: a clinical update. *Internal Medicine Journal*, 50, 24–29.

Hay, P., Bacaltchuk, J., Claudino, A., Ben-Tovim, D., & Yong, P.Y. (2003). Individual psychological therapy in the outpatient treatment of adults with anorexia nervosa. *Cochrane Database System Review*, 4, CD003909.

Insel, T. (2022a). *Healing: Our Path from Mental Illness to Mental Health*. New York: Penguin Press.

Insel, T. (2022b). Quoted in *New York Times*. Sounding an alarm for healing. *Science Times*, February 22, p. D1.

Kagan, J. (1995). On attachment. *Harvard Review of Psychiatry*, 3(2), 104–106.

Kaye, W.H., & Bulik, C.M. (2021). Treatment of patients with anorexia nervosa in the US-a crisis in care. *Journal of the American Medical Association*, 78(6), 591–592.

Lipsitt, L.P. (1977). The study of sensory and learning processes of the newborn. *Clinical Perinatology*, 4(1), 163–186.

Lowe, B., Zipfel, S., Buchholz, C., Dupont, Y., Reas, D.L., & Herzog, W. (2001). Long-term outcome of anorexia nervosa in a prospective 21-year follow-up study. *Psychological Medicine*, 31(5), 881–890.

Madden, S., Miskovic-Wheatley, J., Wallis, A., Kohn, M., Lock, J., LeGrange, D., Jo, B., Clarke, S., Rhodes, P., Hay, P., & Touyz, S. (2015). A randomized controlled trial of in-patient treatment for anorexia nervosa in medically unstable adolescents. *Psychological Medicine*, 45(2), 415–427.

Raju, T.N. (2011). Breastfeeding is a dynamic biological process—not imply a meal at the breast. *Breastfeeding Medicine*, 6, 257–259.

Sawhill, C., Fipps, D.C., Palomo, M.S., & Miller, M. (2020). End-stage anorexia nervosa: when to say "when"—a literature review of an ethically complicated case. *Psychosomatics*, 61(6), 779–786.

Schneiderman, L.J., Jecker, N.S., & Jonsen, A.R. (1990). Medical futility: its meaning and ethical implications. *Annals of Internal Medicine*, 112, 949–954.

Steinhausen, H.C. (2002). The outcome of anorexia nervosa in the 20th century. *American Journal of Psychiatry*, 159(8), 1284–1293.

Vandereycken, W., & Lowenkopf, E.L. (1990). Anorexia nervosa in the 19th century. *Journal of Nervous and Mental Disease*, 178(8), 531–535.

Winnicott, D.W. (1960). The theory of the parent-child relationship. *International Journal of Psychoanalysis*, 41, 585–595.

Winnicott, D.W. (1966). Psycho-somatic illness in its positive and negative aspects. *International Journal of Psychoanalysis*, 47(4), 510–516.

Winnicott, D.W. (1992). *The Child, the Family, and the Outside World*. New York: Perseus Publishing.

Zipfel, S., Giel, K.E., Bulik, C.M., Hay, P., & Schmidt, U. (2015). Anorexia nervosa: aetiology, assessment and treatment. *Lancet Psychiatry*, 2(12), 1099–1111.

Appendix 1
Insights

What have we learned, not only of Ms. B but of anorexia nervosa? The following "insights" come to mind.

1. All cases of anorexia nervosa are unique.
2. There is probably no such thing as a "typical" case.
3. Not all cases "thrive" on "relentless pursuit of thinness."
4. It is difficult, if not impossible, to know exactly what helps patients with anorexia nervosa.
5. It is virtually impossible for therapists working with patients with anorexia to remain totally in control of their own emotions.
6. The urge to prescribe medication usually goes unrewarded.
7. "Insight" is rare in patients with anorexia.
8. Psychoanalytic approaches are rare, seldom advised and often ineffective.
9. General physicians and pediatricians can do better at identifying early signs of eating disorders (see Appendix 2).
10. It is helpful for patient and caretaker to like each other.
11. Diagnosis may be "fluid" depending on what stage of illness is observed. This patient had been seen as having obsessive-compulsive disorder, psychosis, narcissistic character disorder, and borderline personality at different times in her course.
12. Mother attachment in this case and perhaps all cases is pivotal in initiating and sustaining illness.
13. Sexual conflict is a source of struggle between mother and daughter.
14. Hospitalizations (medical) usually involve only refeeding, not psychiatric treatment.
15. Concerns about body image, related to shame, interpersonal relations, and so on, are not prevalent or constant in all cases. (A drawing [see Figure A1.1] reveals personal idealized image, although bodily preoccupation was not prominent.)
16. "Animal therapy" may be an untried potential intervention. (Ms. B finally had her "baby" (cat) until administration disposed of it [shadows of mother!].)

[redacted] 12/4/61

Draw a person
Took about 35 mins.
Painstaking, lots erasures
Hadn't drawn since high schoo
Used to be good at it.
Drew neckline according to
how she remembered old lady
in nightgown in next bed
Trouble with shoes and legs
Said she should have erased
line under hair

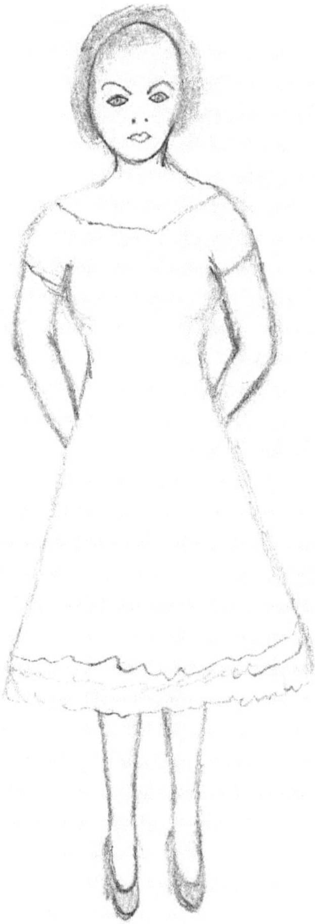

Figure A1.1 Ms. B's response to instruction "draw a picture".

17 It seems unlikely that any of the recent research on causes of anorexia (genetics, endocrinology, brain metabolism, neurosensitivity, microbiome and so on) would have helped Ms. B. But research must persist.
18 Accurate prevalence rates are difficult to obtain but are assumed to be increasing (especially during the pandemic; Marino et al., 2021). Cultural interests in dancing, gymnastics, modelling, acting and others continue to pose a risk for eating disorders, particularly anorexia nervosa.
19 Dieting and dating are a suspicious duo and should alert physicians.
20 Efforts at weight loss or gain seemed related less to a matter of faulty body image or "pursuit of thinness" (the "skinny disease") than to attitudes toward mother and male friends.
21 Memory is not consistent over time.
22 It is very difficult to factor in the impact of anxiety and stress on vacillations in disease.
23 More progress has been made in classifying eating disorders than in identifying etiology of anorexia nervosa (Hay, 2020).

References

Hay, P. (2020). Current approach to eating disorders: a clinical update. *Internal Medicine Journal*, 50, 24–29.

Marino, A., Gliubizzi, C., Reina, F., Nocera, G.M., Marchese, F., & Trapolino, E. (2021). Increase in admissions for anorexia nervosa after lockdown measures: focus on a children's neuropsychiatry unit. *General Hospital Psychiatry*, 72, 147–148.

Appendix 2

Early Detection and Resources

While researchers urgently explore potential answers to the question of etiology, anorexia nervosa and its ravages remain a “crisis.” It is therefore imperative that “frontline” physicians and other health-care professionals, whom patients with evolving eating disorders first consult, be alert to suggestive indicators of impending disease. The following recommendations for general physicians, pediatricians, gynecologists and other primary care clinicians and health-care professionals may help to “catch” markers suggestive of the disease.

1. Welcome patients with an open, interested and receptive demeanor.
2. Do not be over-controlling; let patients talk.
3. Avoid shaming about weight or body “fixations.”
4. Inquire tactfully (not critically) into dieting and dating activities, “secret” or “picky” eating.
5. Record symptoms of gastrointestinal distress (e.g., pain, bloating, distention, nausea, vomiting and constipation).
6. Note presence of anemia.
7. Resist temptation to refer prematurely (unless services of an eating disorders specialist are clearly indicated).
8. Be aware of excessive use of laxatives (or other supplements, etc.).
9. Note dental staining (usually from vomiting).
10. Gently explore mother–daughter (rarely son) relationships.
11. Inquire into hyperactivity of sports, gymnastics and so on.
12. Note distortions of body awareness.
13. Inquire into obsessional behavior, rituals, “habits” and perfectionism.
14. Question sleep habits.
15. Check body hair (lanugo).
16. Explore issues of possible low self-esteem (schoolwork, friends, etc.), depression and suicidal thoughts.
17. Do not wait for patient to make own appointment. Denial is a main feature of the illness. Assign regular return visits.

The following resources are useful:

Further Reading

Fairburn, C.G., Cooper, Z., Doll, H.A., & Davis, B. A. (2005). Identifying dieters who will develop an eating disorder: a prospective, population-based study. *American Journal of Psychiatry*, 162(12), 2249–2255.

Harris, R.T. (1986). Eating disorders: diagnosis and management by the internist. *Southern Medical Journal*, 79(7), 871–878.

Rowe, E. Early detection of eating disorders in general practice. *Australasian Family Physician*, 46(11), 833–838.

Walsh, J.M., Wheat, M.E., & Freund, K. (2000). Detection, evaluation, and treatment of eating disorders: the role of the primary care physician. *Journal of General Internal Medicine*, 15(8), 577–590.

Helpful Resources

National Eating Disorders Association
National Association of Anorexia Nervosa and Associated Disorders
Academy of Eating Disorders
International Association of Eating Disorders
American Psychiatric Association (guidelines for eating disorders)

Appendix 3
Correspondence regarding Ms. B

Dec. 5, 1962

Dr. Felix Deutsch
44 Larchwood Rd.
Cambridge, Mass.

Dear Doctor Deutsch:

I thought you might be interested in hearing about a patient you saw many years ago at the Beth Israel Hospital. Her name is [redacted] and her case history appears in your 1939 paper on The Associative Anamnesis as well as in the 1940 paper on Anorexia Nervosa (with Waller and Kaufman).

I first met [redacted] in the Emergency Ward, where she was brought over 1 year ago in a stuporous state. A diagnosis of "catatonia" was made by the house officer and I was called for psychiatric consultation. I thought she was suffering from something organic in addition to her emotional difficulties and suggested that she be admitted to the B.I. rather than sent to Boston State Hospital as had been requested. Just before being sent upstairs to the ward, she had a grand mal seizure and about 30 minutes after arriving on the ward, had a massive hematemesis which nearly exsanguinated her. Repeated transfusions and a long hospital convalescence helped her recovery and I have followed her intermittently since that time. It is of great interest to note that her personality structure is essentially unchanged from your early description and on psychological tests she appears more like a severe obsessive-compulsive, even though her social adjustment is indeed, for all practical purposes, a psychotic one.

In my scan of the literature on anorexia nervosa, I have not found a single case reported with a 25-year follow-up and feel that this case report would be an important contribution to the literature, in view of your historic connection with the case as well as its follow-up significance. I am presently writing up the case and would feel highly honored if, after the case is written, you would be willing to add some comments of your own to the report. At any rate, I shall send you a full report of the case when I have completed it.

Sincerely yours,

Don R. Lipsitt, M.D.

Figure A3.1 Letter from Dr. Lipsitt to Dr. Felix Deutsch, December 5, 1962.

FELIX DEUTSCH
44 LARCHWOOD DRIVE
CAMBRIDGE 38. MASS.

UNIVERSITY
4-6244

December 10, 1962.

Dr. Don R. Lipsitt
Beth Israel Hospital
330 Brookline Avenue
Boston 15, Mass.

Dear Dr. Lipsitt:

I am looking forward with great interest to your report regarding [redacted] whose name I had forgotten. I shall communicate with Dr. Kaufman before discussing further this case.

Thank you for your co-operation.

Sincerely yours,

Felix Deutsch

FELIX DEUTSCH, M.D.

FD:eb

Figure A3.2 Letter from Dr. Deutsch to Dr. Lipsitt, December 10, 1962.

The University of New Mexico

School of Medicine
Mental Health Programs
Department of Psychiatry
2400 Tucker, NE
Albuquerque, NM 87131
Telephone (505) 277-2223

February 15, 1990

Donald Oken, M.D.
Editor-in-Chief, Psychosomatic Medicine
Department of Psychiatry
Pennsylvania Hospital
Philadelphia, Pennsylvania 19107

<u>LETTER TO THE EDITOR</u>

Dear Dr. Oken,

In his article in the 50th anniversary issue of Psychosomatic Medicine (Vol II, 597-607, 1989) Don Lipsett pays tribute to Felix Deutsch as one of the first analysts to make a significant contribution to psychosomatic medicine. That Felix Deutsch deserves such recognition there can be no doubt , since this is evident from one of his earliest papers (1).

Lipsett cites Alexander and Selesnick who stated that Felix Deutsch and Georg Groddeck were "the most consistent proponents of the significance of emotional factors, not only in hysterical conversion symptoms but also in chronic disease"(1). However Alexander and Selesnick also stated that Felix Deutsch and Georg Groddeck "uncritically attempted to explain all symptoms as the direct expression of highly repressed ideas of fantasies" and furthermore Deutsch "applied Freud's concept of conversion to all dysfunctions of the body" (3). That there is justification in Alexander's criticism is evidenced from Deutsch's writing long after 1939. In 1955 he wrote "the treatment of any psychosomatic disorder is to purify and liberate the bodily functions from their unconscious cathexis" (4). In discussing epilepsy he wrote that "convulsive seizures represent the gratification of hostile or aggressive tendencies...in the seizures the sado-masochistic tendencies are acted out" (5). The idea of giving meaning to seizures was negated some years before Deutsch's chapter on epilepsy (6). Lipsett does mention

A Place in Your Future

Figure A3.3 Letter from Dr. Rosenbaum to Dr. Oken, February 15, 1990.

Deutsch's "emphasis on the role of symbolization in the etiology and course of illness" but lauds it "as landmark efforts to go beyond mere descriptive reductionistic approaches to diagnosis and treatment".

I cite Alenxander's criticism with which I agree, since I believe they are pertinent to the case report which is the vehicle Lipsett uses to illustrate Deutsch's contribution to psychosomatic medicine.

The patient with anorexia nervosa whose case is beautifully presented by Lipsett was first seen by Deutsch in 1938 and by Lipsett in 1961 and then followed by him until the present. In reviewing the chart at the time of the admission when the patient was seen by Deutsch, Lipsett was impressed by Deutsch's words "that no improvement can be hoped for until this patient is given insight and placed in an environment removed from the mother". Lipsett endows these words as prophetic since after the patient's mother died in 1968 she was placed in a nursing home where she remains to this very day.

I too would endow the words as prophetic but I see them as a self-fulfilling prophesy since they may have been responsible for instituting a course of treatment that was doomed to failure. In my opinion the one thing the patient did not need was analytically oriented insight therapy, which was given in abundance. Also the order "to be removed from the mother" was probably responsible for the attempts by various therapists to separate the patient and her mother which only aggravated the problem. It should have been clear from the start that only death could separate such an intense symbiotic relationship.

I believe that not only in retrospect, but in 1938 some analytically oriented clinicians would not have recommended insight therapy, nor encouraged attempts to separate the patient and her mother. Rather, the therapy then, and for a similar case today, would be long-term relationship therapy preferably with a woman therapist, perhaps a social worker. By long-term I mean that the therapist must accept the fact that taking on such a patient is a life-long commitment for both patient and therapist. In such a therapeutic situation the patient and her mother probably would not have been physically separated during the mother's lifetime but it might have given the patient a chance to live a more productive life rather than continue the symbiotic relationship with mother substitutes in a nursing home for these past 22 years.

At the time Deutsch saw this patient in 1938 he was also on the staff of the Massachusetts General Hospital where I knew him since I was a resident in psychiatry. In contrast to Deutsch's approach Eric Lindeman, also on the staff and also an analyst, saw a patient, an adolescent of 16 with a severe attack of ulcerative colitis. The patient had an older brother to whom he

Figure A3.3 (Continued)

was closely attached and who was very protective of his fragile younger brother. The attack of ulcerative colitis broke out when the older brother left for the Army. The analytically oriented prescription was to replace the brother by selecting a therapist for the patient a brother substitute, i.e. a young male social worker. This maneuver together with good medical care was successful. Obviously no one can say that any type of therapeutic intervention would have helped Lipsett's patient bu in my opinion if she were seen today she would not be given the prescription of 1938.

Since Lipsett's article was one of several celebrating the 50th anniversary of "Psychosomatic Medicine" I just want to add the names of Stanley Cobb and Franz Alexander, both of whom were on the first Editorial Board of the Journal, as two of the truly greats in the history of psychosomatic medicine in the United States. Only a Stanley Cobb could have started a dynamically oriented psychiatric inpatient unit at the Massachusetts Genera in 1934 and invited outstanding psychoanalytic refugees, including the Deutschs, to become members of the faculty and hospital staff. In addition to his well-known achievements in psychosomatic medicine, Franz Alexander also founded the only major psychoanalytic institute in this country that has not split since its founding in 1931. The main reason for this, I believe, is that Franz Alexander, academically and scientifically oriented, created a truly academic atmosphere in that institute which tolerated differences of opinions rather than excommunicating non-believers and thereby causing splits and new institutes.

With best wishes for the continued success of the Journal.

Sincerely,

Milton Rosenbaum M.D

Milton Rosenbaum, M.D.
Visiting Professor

Figure A3.3 (Continued)

PSYCHOSOMATIC MEDICINE

Journal of the American Psychosomatic Society

Editorial Office: Department of Psychiatry, Pennsylvania Hospital
8th and Spruce Streets, Philadelphia, PA 19107
215-829-5581

February 27, 1990

Don R. Lipsitt, M.D.
Mount Auburn Hospital
330 Mount Auburn Street
Cambridge, MA 02238

Dear Don,

As you know, we occasionally print "Letters to the Editor", when someone writes in about an article we have published. In such instances, I offer the original author the opportunity to write a response which I then publish with the incoming letter.

Attached is a letter just received from Milt Rosenbaum about your article on Felix Deutsch, etc. It came as a surprise, both because it would never occur to me that someone would write in response to an historical article in a commemorative issue, and because I did not realize that Milt was still active. (To be an Editor is to be surprised constantly by others' behavior!)

Were the letter from anyone other than a person like Milt, probably I wouldn't consider publishing it. However, as he is, in a way, sort of a historical figure, himself, I am inclined to do so. Do you have any problem with this?

If I do go ahead with it, do you feel you want to write a "response" for publication? My advice to you would be not to do so. It isn't necessary either for the record nor to rescue Deutsch's reputation, which certainly is secure; and it strikes me as a bit unseemly to be squabbling over the latter.

When you get the chance, telephone and let me know what you'd like to do.

Cordially,

Don

Donald Oken, M.D.
Editor-in-Chief

DO:ibm

Figure A3.4 Letter from Dr. Oken to Dr. Lipsitt, February 27, 1990.

UNIVERSITY OF
ROCHESTER
MEDICAL CENTER

STRONG MEMORIAL HOSPITAL
SCHOOL OF MEDICINE AND DENTISTRY
SCHOOL OF NURSING

ans. 10/23/90

John Romano, M.D.
Distinguished University Professor
of Psychiatry, Emeritus

October 9, 1990

Don R. Lipsitt, M.D.
Department of Psychiatry
Mt. Auburn Hospital
330 Mt. Auburn Street
Cambridge, MA 02238

Dear Dr. Lipsitt:

After reading with interest your paper entitled, "Anorexia Nervosa, Felix Deutsch, and the Associative Anamnesis: A Psychosomatic Kaleidoscope," published in Psychosomatic Medicine, November-December 1989, and the exchange of letters between you and Milton Rosenbaum which followed, I had the opportunity to discuss your paper with Milton on the occasion of his 80th birthday party which was held at his home in Augusta, Kentucky, early in September of this year. You may not know that my friendship with Milt goes back to 1938 when I served as a Rockefeller Fellow in Neurology at the Boston City Hospital when he was a psychiatric resident at McLean Hospital. In 1942, when I was appointed professor and chairman of the Department of Psychiatry in Cincinnati, Milt Rosenbaum was my remarkably able associate as we worked together during the War years and before I left Cincinnati for Rochester (1946

The principal reason I am writing you is that the patient, [redacted], about whom you write was also my patient at the Peter Bent Brigham, where I served from 1939 to 1942 before I went to Cincinnati. I am sending you copies of notes about [redacted] and her mother. This is not a copy of the hospital record, which I do not have, but I suppose if you wished to see it, you could find it at the Brigham. I was most interested to learn about your experiences with th patient in 1961 and now in her 70's when you met with her in the nursing home in which she lives. As you indicate in your comments, she presented many interesting problems in diagnosis, including the explanation of her yellowness which was found to be due to carotinemia from eating large amounts of carrots and parsley. At one time, the patient told me that she felt better when she w thin and yellow than when she was fat and white. During the reversal of her sleep pattern, she would spend much of the time sitting on the toilet, at time eating bananas, and quite often, she would interrupt the sleep of her parents by coming into their bedroom and inserting her clothes between her father's and mother's clothes in the closet.

Milt Rosenbaum, as well as Franz Alexander, were more charitable in their comments about Felix Deutsch than I am. In 1939, I was appointed a Sigmund Freud Fellow in Psychoanalysis at the Boston Psychoanalytic Institute together with Charles Brenner and George Gardner. In the years that followed,

300 Crittenden Boulevard
Rochester, New York 14642
(716) 275-3047

Figure A3.5 Letter from Dr. Romano to Dr. Lipsitt, October 9, 1990.

Don R. Lipsitt, M.D. -2- October 9, 1990

I attended most of the seminars as well as the special lectures given by members of the Psychoanalytic Institute staff. The remarks made by Felix Deutsch at many of these conferences were not only lacking in substance, but were for the most part exaggerated notions of cause and effect. I remember vividly several times when his outrageous remarks held no relevance to the case history material presented by the lecturer.

With Milt, I would also pay tribute to Stanley Cobb and to Franz Alexander for their initial and pioneering contributions to the field. While I am at it, I would also like to pay tribute to my old and dearest friend, Milt Rosenbaum, who, I believe, is one of the outstanding psychiatric clinicians of our time.

Sincerely yours,

JR:rmf
cc: Milton Rosenbaum, M.D.
Enclosures

P.S.: I am also including some brief notes on a seminar conducted at the Boston Psychoanalytic Institute in December 1941 in which [redacted] is mentioned briefly, and in which you will find a note indicating that Dr. Tartakoff said that [redacted] was currently (December 1941) at the Boston Psychopathic Hospital.

P.P.S.: If you should visit [redacted] again, would you be kind enough to tell her that I remember her vividly and that I wish her good things in her life. She probably will not remember me.

P.P.P.S.: I am sending a copy of this material to Milt Rosenbaum.

Figure A3.5 (Continued)

MARSHALL UNIVERSITY
DEPARTMENT OF PSYCHIATRY
School of Medicine
Huntington, West Virginia 25755-9460
304/696-7077

Dr. L. Lipsitt
Editor
Gen. Hosp. Psych.

Nov 2-1990

re "Violence on Psychiatric Wards – Role of Psy Ray Milieu"

Dear Don –

In regard to the letter from Ex. Ed. of "General Hospital Psychiatry" concerning the Fig. for my article above I am enclosing a photographic copy of the Fig.

John Romano sent me the copy of your letter to him re the case of "[redacted]". What an amazing co-incidence. I imagine she is the only pt. with "Anorexia Nervosa" followed for this long a period.

Another interesting aspect of the case is that she resembles

A STATE UNIVERSITY OF WEST VIRGINIA

Figure A3.6 Letter from Dr. Rosenbaum to Dr. Lipsitt, November 2, 1990.

2

MARSHALL UNIVERSITY

DEPARTMENT OF PSYCHIATRY
School of Medicine
Huntington, West Virginia 25755-9460
304/696-7077

the kind of pt with dx of "anorexia nervosa" I used to see many many years ago. They were all "psychotic" - and looked like schizophrenics - yet were not schizophrenic - but they certainly were "crazy" - not like the cases today.

I'm looking forward to seeing you at the Psycho-Som. Soc. Meeting in Santa Fe in March -- I am scheduled to lead a luncheon group on the subject of "Relationship of Consultation Psych. to Psycho-Somatic Medicine"

Warmest greetings

Milt Rosenbaum

A STATE UNIVERSITY OF WEST VIRGINIA

Figure A3.6 (Continued)

Index

Note: Page numbers in *italics* refer to figures.

For Product Safety Concerns and Information please contact our EU
representative GPSR@taylorandfrancis.com
Taylor & Francis Verlag GmbH, Kaufingerstraße 24, 80331 München, Germany

www.ingramcontent.com/pod-product-compliance
Ingram Content Group UK Ltd.
Pitfield, Milton Keynes, MK11 3LW, UK
UKHW022313250926
475702UK00046B/766
* 9 7 8 1 0 3 2 0 7 7 6 7 3 *